Therapeutic Thematic Arts Programming
for Older Adults

A portion of the author's earnings from sales of this book will be donated to the Levine Madori Single Parent Scholarship Fund at the American Therapeutic Recreation Association.
Visit http://www.atra-tr.org

Therapeutic Thematic Arts Programming

for Older Adults

by

Linda Levine Madori, Ph.D., CTRS, ATR-BC

St. Thomas Aquinas College
Sparkill, New York

4/08

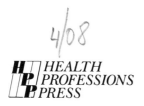

**HEALTH
PROFESSIONS
PRESS**

Baltimore • London • Sydney

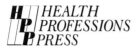

Health Professions Press, Inc.
Post Office Box 10624
Baltimore, Maryland 21285-0624

www.healthpropress.com

TTAP™ is a trademark of Linda Levine Madori.

Art on the cover and pp. xii, 6, 24, 36, 58, 84, and 102 © 2006 Linda Levine Madori.

Typeset by Maryland Composition Co., Inc., Glen Burnie, Maryland.
Manufactured in the United States of America by
Sheridan Books, Inc., Chelsea, Michigan.

The information provided in this book is in no way meant to substitute for a medical practitioner's advice or expert opinion. Readers should consult a medical professional if they are interested in more information. This book is sold without warranties of any kind, express or implied, and the publisher and author disclaim any liability, loss, or damage caused by the contents of this book.

Library of Congress Cataloging-in-Publication Data

Levine Madori, Linda.
  Therapeutic thematic arts programming for older adults / by Linda Levine Madori.
     p.   cm.
  Includes bibliographical references and index.
  ISBN-13: 978-1-932529-02-9 (pbk.)
  ISBN-10: 1-932529-02-0 (pbk.)
  1. Art therapy.   2. Older people—Mental health.   I. Title.
  [DNLM: 1. Art Therapy.   2. Aged.   WM 450.5.A8 L665t 2005]
  RC489.A7L475   2007
  616.89'1656–dc22   2006020016

British Library Cataloguing in Publication data are available from the British Library.

Contents

About the Author

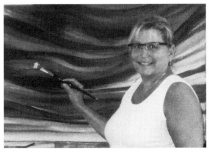

For the last 25 years, Linda Levine Madori, Ph.D., CTRS, ATR-BC has worked in the field of gerontology and dementia-specific services and research including designing innovative creative arts programming for well elderly, assisted living, skilled nursing, senior housing, and other long-term care settings. Currently she is researching the effects of the Therapeutic Thematic Arts Programming (TTAP) Method with individuals in New York who have mild Alzheimer's disease.

Since 1991, Dr. Levine Madori has presented more than 100 papers on the arts and aging. She has lectured extensively in Spain, Switzerland, Indonesia, Lithuania, Czech Republic, Russia, China, Italy, and the United States. She has chaired the Leisure Track of the American Society on Aging, developed professional intensives for the American Art Therapy Association, and developed and implemented educational workshops and professional panel presentations for educators and psychologists as an Ambassador Leader for the People to People International educational program.

Dr. Levine Madori is an associate professor at St. Thomas Aquinas College in Sparkill, New York, where she has taught therapeutic recreation and creative arts therapies since 1996. Her dissertation research in Alzheimer's disease, cognition, and psychosocial well-being is the basis for *Therapeutic Thematic Arts Programming for Older Adults*. This book will be followed by the *TTAP Method for Alzheimer's* and the *TTAP Method for Caregivers of Alzheimer's Disease*.

Awarded a Senior Specialist Fulbright scholarship, Dr. Levine Madori was invited to teach the TTAP Method and lecture at Waikato University in Auckland, New Zealand, and Victoria University in Melbourne, Australia in 2007. She will also speak at the Alzheimer's New Zealand national conference in Wellington regarding the significance of art and brain wellness.

Dr. Levine Madori is an avid artist and painter, and the paintings shown on the chapter dividers are her own work.

Contact Dr. Levine Madori regarding how you have used this new method or other questions at Linda@Levinemadoriphd.com.

Acknowledgments

A very special thank you goes to my publisher, Mary Magnus, for her enthusiastic support and for believing in me and my work before I really did; to my editor, Janet Krejci, for her keen sense of knowing exactly what I wanted to express; and to Dr. William Wargo for his strong belief in my work and his compassion and wit that got me through an entire year. I am also grateful to my dissertation advisors who believed in my academic research pursuits and encouraged me to continue writing: Dr. R. Malgady, Dr. E. Mitty, and Dr. A. Grossman.

I would like to thank two individuals who, unbeknownst to me at the time, directly affected my professional development by encouraging my further education: Maria Scaros Mercado, LCAT, DMT, and Dr. Susan Marell, Professor of Psychology and Director of the Honors Program at St. Thomas Aquinas College.

To my four children, Lorin, Lea, Melanie, and Casey, I am profoundly grateful for all the love and joy you bring to my life, which kept me going all those days and nights working on my laptop at the kitchen table.

My gratitude goes to all those older adults, over the past 25 years, whom I had the pleasure to meet and with whom I had the opportunity to work by introducing the creative arts into their lives.

To all my students at St. Thomas Aquinas College, who have graduated and become my peers; you filled my classes, questioned my thought processes and theoretical beliefs, and responded enthusiastically to all that I taught—a big thank you.

A special acknowledgment goes to my closest and dearest friends who have, over time, continually given me their love and support and have become a part of my family: Bobbi Vogel, Leonor Linares, and Linda Cimillo.

To my husband, Lee David Auerbach, Esq., who brought me through the dissertation process and the writing of this book by being my mentor, best friend, and computer expert. Lee, you continually listened to all my concerns, you came to my rescue whenever needed, and gently guided me to grow into all that I am today. I am forever grateful, and please, never stop counting the days until our next vacation!

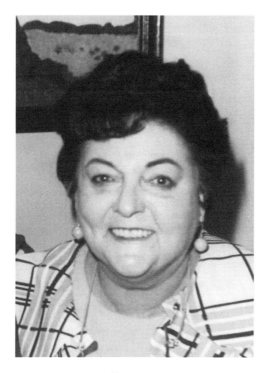

Mary Ellen Reilly Levine
(Grandma Betty)

This book is dedicated to the memory of Grandma Betty, whose
unconditional love changed my life in more ways than I can count.
She continues to live on today, through stories and photographs
that are shared with my own four children.
Through her unconditional support and guidance, I recognize her
reflection in each individual with whom I have worked
and each life I have influenced.
This book is a tribute to her life then, now, and beyond,
for she continues to inspire me.
I will always carry her in my heart, for her love gives me
a great sense of joy and peace.

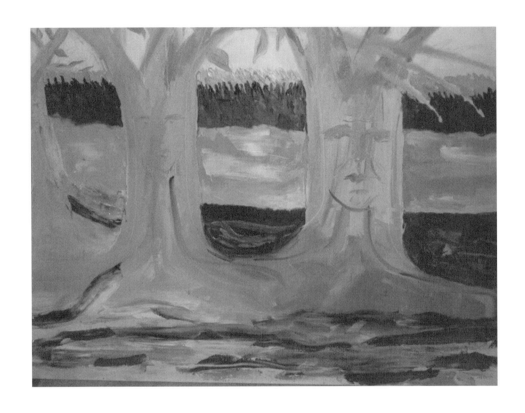

Introduction

The foundations of this book come from more than 25 years of the author's hands-on experience in working with older adults as a Certified Recreation Therapist and a Board-Certified Art Therapist. The Therapeutic Thematic Arts Programming (TTAP™) method is an enjoining of the principles of therapeutic recreation and the creative arts therapies into a singular technique for therapists who work with older adults at all stages in the continuum of elder care, including community services for well elderly, rehabilitation programs, assisted living facilities, skilled nursing care, and services for Alzheimer's disease. The TTAP method is based on new research that has enhanced the understanding of the connection between how humans learn physiologically and how humans age developmentally, thereby enabling therapists to develop and facilitate more biologically effective, time-efficient, and creative programming for what is fast becoming the largest special group of the 21st century: older adults.

The TTAP method has five main objectives:

1. To embrace the concept of *use it or lose it* by stimulating all areas of brain functioning to enhance cognitive, emotional, physical, and social capacity

2. To provide opportunities for the individual to integrate life experiences into group experiences through object relations in the creative arts process

3. To provide a system in which the individual can reintegrate into a supportive social group to foster feelings of safety and support and thereby increase social participation

4. To engage the participant in a multitude of creative arts experiences: music, drawing, sculpture, movement, poetry, and special theme events

5. To provide programming that enables the *flow* to flourish

Chapter 1 offers an overview of the current research on brain growth, development, and cell regrowth. Case studies from the late 20th century to the beginning of the 21st century provide a stimulating new understanding of how brain functioning can be enhanced through therapeutic activities that use both the right and the left hemispheres of the brain. The TTAP method reflects this new understanding of brain functioning in a nine-step method that integrates and stimulates various areas of the brain through a variety of specific therapeutic activities. This chapter also reviews current research on the physiology of the brain (the motor cortex, the sensory cortex, the parietal lobe, the occipital lobe, the cerebellum, the brain stem, reticular formation, Wernicke's area, the temporal lobe, and Broca's area) and how the brain processes memory and language as well as learning and intelligence. In Bloom's six stages of learning, knowledge and how humans understand through recall of previously learned information and/ or tasks are discussed in relation to how the therapist can use recall in the interactive creative arts experience. Understanding that individuals comprehend information differently validates and gives reason to approaching the therapeutic experience using varying learning styles, an inherent feature of the TTAP. Examples illustrate how the therapist can increase his or her understanding of the group dynamics through TTAP. Also discussed is how analysis, synthesis, and evaluation of learning are basic concepts on which the TTAP method is based. In addition, Chapter 1 explains how three systems of the brain—the recognition system, the strategic system, and the affective system—are applied and used in the TTAP method.

Chapter 2 discusses two distinct areas that are the theoretical underpinnings of the TTAP method: theories on aging that stress the importance of activities throughout the life span and the theoretical framework on which therapeutic recreation was founded. The theories of aging first are explored from a humanistic perspective in developmental theory and lifespan theory. These theories explain why people do what they do and are the theoretical structures out of which the TTAP method has grown. Through the understanding of the theoretical framework also comes the understanding of why and how the TTAP method naturally creates a structure in which the therapist can facilitate self-determination, self-efficacy, optimal experiences, and a sense of overall well-being, which are discussed in detail in Chapter 3.

Chapter 3 provides a history of therapeutic recreation and examines and analyzes how the TTAP method facilitates activities that provide opportunities for development of self-esteem, self-development, and self-awareness through self-expression in the creative arts. TTAP is a structured way to incorporate and stimulate the three systems of the brain while developing and implementing therapeutic recreation activities. Some of the benefits of TTAP that are discussed include the following:

- Provides a natural way of learning and processing information through activities

- Offers the participants a deep understanding of the subject or topic

- Is structured yet flexible and is individualized for each participant's learning needs or interests

- Incorporates all creative arts therapies to complement the therapeutic process

- Establishes a flow between each activity

- Can incorporate broad subject matter to allow for brainstorming within a structured yet flexible environment

- Can provide significant relevance to real life

A significant goal of the TTAP method is to allow the participant to experience all types of creative art, including music, movement, writing, sculpture, movement and music combined, poetry, culinary activities, theme events, and photography. These nine types of creative art are the foundation of the nine steps of TTAP and are discussed in depth in Chapter 4. Three main goals are woven into the TTAP method:

1. To identify a fundamental link among self-esteem, self-worth, and intrinsic motivation and encourage this process to take place continually within the group through the ongoing use of creativity

2. To elevate each individual's self-expression to a central position in all programming through the continual use of past and present personal pursuits, life experiences, and interests that have accrued across the life span

3. To develop each individual's unique combination of skills, multiple intelligences, and capabilities for self-expression by using individual activities and cooperative groups and stimulating multiple perspectives

Chapter 5 discusses the Continuum of Psychological Domains and how it expands on the Accountability Model of Service (Stumbo & Peterson, 2004) to develop activities that best meet the social, emotional, cognitive, physical, and spiritual needs of the individual at each stage of wellness. The TTAP method focuses on the overall enhancement of the leisure function but also addresses the individual's specific needs in five domains related to where he or she is along the health spectrum of aging, allowing for customized programming directly to their needs. These five domains can be analyzed in each area of aging: well elderly, assisted living, skilled nursing, cognitive impairment, and hospice care. Individuals in various areas of health care have different needs in each domain, and each individual can have different needs within that special group. Furthermore, each domain can be targeted by programming, and the chosen theme can focus on a specific psychological need. This approach has never been taken before in developing therapeutic recreation for older adults. Through the use of TTAP, therefore, the therapist can assess where along the Continuum of Psychological Domains each individual falls and develop programming that best meets the individual's needs at various points throughout the continuum. Most important, the therapist can develop programming that is designed specifically for the emotional, social, physical, or cognitive benefit of the individual at that particular moment. There is a TTAP assessment form in Appendix B.

Chapter 6 discusses how the Continuum of Psychological Domains is used in each area of aging care, including assisted living, rehabilitation, skilled nursing care, and Alzheimer's care. It provides specific examples of how each of the nine steps of TTAP can be tailored to meet the needs of these varied groups of older adults. In addition, a detailed overview of Alzheimer's disease is provided.

The 21st century has started off with great new discoveries in the workings of the various areas of the brain as a result of modern advances in medicine and technology. The brain can be examined for the first time while a person is alive and well. Scientists can see brain activity in the neurons through positron emission tomography emulsion scans, computerized axial tomography scans, and other noninvasive methods while a person is at rest or engaging in an activity. This was virtually impossible in the early 1990s. Eastern and western medicine both suggest that physiological connections exist among body, mind, and spirit. Brain research now has revealed that continual stimulation of memory, both short and long term, plays an integral role in the wellness of the brain and, thus, in overall quality of life. Research is demonstrating a high correlation between creative processes and decreased heart rate, increased brain activity in specific pleasure areas of the brain, and an overall sense of well-being.

This book is intended to bring a new body of knowledge to the field of creative arts therapy to assist therapists in better assessing, implementing, developing, planning, and evaluating the therapeutic process with the assistance of the TTAP method. It is recommended for the professional therapist who is teaching or practicing; for the instructor who is teaching in creative arts therapy; for the student in creative arts therapy and/or therapeutic recreation; and for the sibling, parent, or friend who needs direction with what to do with an older parent who is well or has some dementia. This new approach in program planning is designed specifically for therapists who work with the largest special group ever to exist: older adults. The more that therapists understand about the physiological, psychological, and social needs of individuals, the better they can provide therapeutic recreation through the use of creative arts therapies.

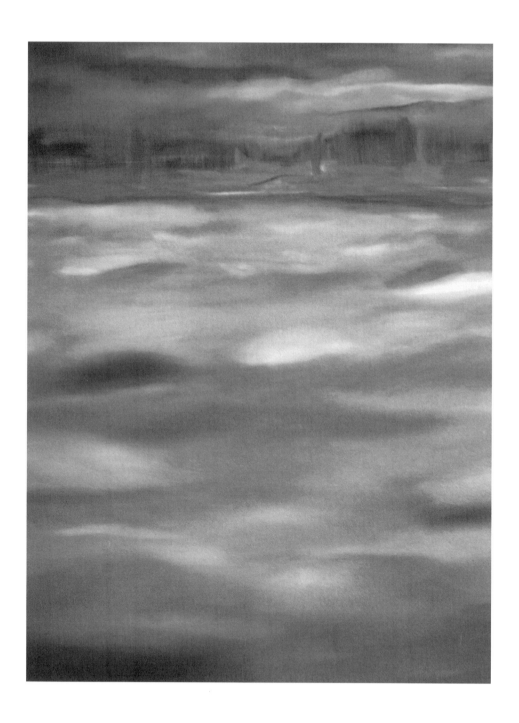

CHAPTER 1

Therapeutic Thematic Arts Programming and Brain Functioning

*To look into our hearts is not
enough.... One must look into
the cerebral cortex.*
—T.S. Eliot

Recent scientific understanding of the brain has been compared with humans' limited understanding of the infinite possibilities of outer space. New research, however, is opening the doors to new understandings of how to stimulate the brain and enhance its functioning. The Therapeutic Thematic Arts Programming (TTAP) method incorporates this new information on how the brain functions into a nine-step method that integrates and stimulates different areas of the brain through a variety of specific therapeutic activities. This chapter reviews current research on how the brain functions, the physiology of the brain, memory and language, and learning and intelligence. The foundations of the TTAP method are explained in relation to current research on brain functioning.

CURRENT RESEARCH ON BRAIN FUNCTION

The 1990s were considered the *decade of the brain* because more was learned about brain function in those 10 years than ever before. Modern technology has enabled the discovery of new facts that alter and forever change concepts concerning how the brain functions that were until these discoveries deemed fact. Child development research before 1990 subscribed to the belief that humans are born with a finite number of brain cells and that, throughout the life span, these cells slowly die off. This basic belief has been wholly disproved since the end of the 1990s. The first attempts to understand the brain were made in the 1960s by a research team at the

University of California, Berkeley. This research, conducted by Dr. Mark Rosenzweig and Dr. Marion Diamond (Diamond, 1999), has proved that the brain can make new cells when stimulated by visual, auditory, sensory, verbal, and/or kinesthetic stimuli. The first research experiment divided a group of very young, genetically linked laboratory mice into two groups. One group of mice was placed into much larger cages with visual and kinesthetic manipulative items, such as wheels, toys, and colorful objects, that were changed weekly to reinforce the enriched environment that encouraged the mice to experiment and interact daily with the new stimuli. The second group of mice was placed in small cages without any toys or stimulation. After 1 year, both groups' brains were weighed, measured, and compared in size and mass. The findings proved for the first time a direct correlation between outside stimulation and brain mass and density. The mice with the enriched environment had more nerve connections and higher levels of neurotransmitters as a result of the constant mental stimulation. The mice that had received no external stimulation had decreased mass and significantly lower levels of neurotransmitters.

While the research at Berkeley continued, new findings were being published by a research team at the University of Illinois (Golomb, Kluger, & de Leon, 1996). These findings confirmed that mentally active mice developed brains that not only were packed more densely with neurons but they also took less time to solve problems, such as learning how to find their way through a maze. The mice with no stimulation showed delayed responses and physical differences in brain mass.

Diamond (1999) found in her continued research at Berkeley that there was biological evidence of the correlation between brain mass and density and education. Studies on 300 randomly donated brains revealed that three distinct thicknesses in the cortex wall exist. Further investigation into the lifestyles of the individuals whose brains had been donated led to a significant scientific discovery: Individuals with less than secondary education had the thinnest wall mass; those who had completed high school and then obtained unskilled jobs had the second thickest wall mass; and those who had completed high school and then gone on to higher education or technical positions had the most dense brain mass. Diamond (1999) discussed in the findings that even occupations that do not necessarily require higher education, such as carpentry, were believed to result in thick cortex walls because of the continual thinking, choice making, and problem solving that are required in these professions.

These findings showed for the first time that an individual's lifestyle has an effect on brain mass, thereby confirming that the brain is able to grow new cells and refuting the previous belief that humans are born with a finite number of brain cells that slowly die off as a person ages. It is this now-refuted notion that underpins the common belief that age is related directly to senility.

Yankner (2000) stated that modern medicine, through technological breakthroughs, is developing new understanding of the brain's functioning and its ability to regrow cells in the hippocampal region. When the brain receives external stimulation, such as reading, writing, and environmental cues, it causes the cells in this region to rejuvenate and reproduce. Medical breakthroughs such as this could affect dramatically how people understand the importance of therapeutic activities throughout the life span as these relate to and directly affect *brain wellness* (Diamond, 1999). Therapists must start to incorporate this understanding into how they provide programming so that it better enhances brain functioning in the individuals whom they are assisting; that is, they must be aware of the importance of continuous sensory stimulation in all therapeutic programming.

The most significant findings to date that support and complement the findings of earlier research come from a study that was started in 1986 at the University of Kentucky: the Nun Study. Snowdon has been studying 678 nuns, all of whom are members of a convent in Minnesota, since they were 16 years of age (Lemonick & Park, 2001). All studied to become teachers. Their personal and medical histories have been researched, they have participated in testing of their cognitive abilities, and their brains have been studied upon their deaths. In his book *Aging with Grace,* Snowdon (2001) revealed significant links between lifestyle in well elderly individuals and the nuns who eventually developed senility, which today is known as Alzheimer's disease (AD).

Snowdon's findings show that a history of stroke or head trauma can increase the probability of developing some form of dementia or AD and that a college education and an active intellectual life may protect a person from the effects of dementia. The autobiographical information that the nuns had written was studied for detail, expression of thought, and complexity of idea. One of the surprising results is that "the way we express ourselves in language, even at an early age, can foretell how long we'll live and how vulnerable we are to getting the disease decades down the line." The National Institute on Aging provided Snowdon with more than $5 million in funding to be used during a 15-year period to research further this "innovative and pioneering study" (Lemonick & Park, 2001, p. 64).

McClellan (2001) published the first research study that examined how specific regions of the brain respond to visual stimulation. He used projected slide images, which were shown to three different groups. These groups, however, had one element in common: They all had diagnosed addictions. The first group comprised alcoholics, the second group comprised cocaine addicts, and the third group comprised food addicts. While all three groups underwent magnetic resonance imaging (MRI), they were shown simultaneously the same 300 photographic images in a theater setting. All participants registered *pleasurable stimulation responses* to specific photographic images; each group responded to the same types of photographs. For example, all of the alcoholics' pleasure sensors were visually stimulated and recorded on the MRI when the images of bar scenes, the

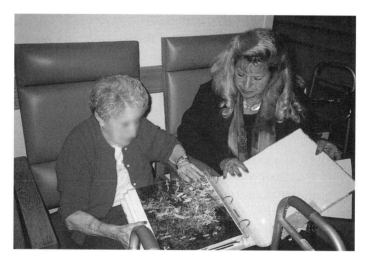

Figure 1.1.   A therapist is visually stimulating while verbally engaging an individual through looking at photographs in a Look Book (copyright © 2004 by L. Levine Madori).

serving of alcoholic beverages, and consumption of alcoholic drinks were viewed. The cocaine addicts' pleasure zones showed stimulation only when photographic images of cocaine, drugs being smoked, or drugs being prepared for consumption were viewed. The food addicts responded only to photographic images of food being eaten or prepared for consumption.

The research findings described in this chapter aid in assembling the puzzle pieces of how the mind works and how to provide better quality thematic programming that incorporates brain stimulation and visual, auditory, and sensory stimulation. It is a logical conclusion from this research that photo therapy, or the use of reminiscence and photographic images, for example, can have a profound effect on the pleasure centers of the brain (see Figure 1.1). An overall sense of well-being can be generated through the use of photographic images, whether printed, projected, or viewed as a film. The core of these research findings is the realization that the more stimulation the brain receives, the better it functions.

DEMENTIA (ALZHEIMER'S DISEASE) AND THE BRAIN

AD was first identified by the German psychiatrist Alois Alzheimer in 1906. In his time, at the beginning of the 20th century, the average life expectancy was 47 years; therefore, most people died young enough to avoid this late-life disease. Since the turn of the last century, however, life expectancy has risen dramatically (from 47 years to 77 years in the United States); as a result, AD has become more prevalent (U.S. Census Bureau, 1997). Approximately 4.5 million Americans—more than one in five of those age 75–84 and nearly half of those age 85 and older—now have AD. The National Alzheimer's Association estimates that six million people will have this disease by 2010, 6.8 million by 2020, 8.7 million by 2030,

11.8 million by 2040, and 14.3 million by 2050. These numbers reflect only those who will have this disease; the number of people who are affected indirectly, such as relatives, spouses, and caregivers, is staggering.

AD is caused by the deterioration of brain cells. A characteristic collection of protein-based plaques and tangles accumulates around these cells. The disorder typically progresses through four stages: mild, moderate, severe, and terminal. In the first stage—mild—one experiences mild memory loss, inability to remember short-term events, and difficulty with engaging in prolonged and detailed verbal conversations. In the second stage—moderate—the individual shows signs of continued social withdrawal and significant cognitive impairment; the person moves from independence to dependence with daily living tasks such as dressing, bathing, eating, and shopping for one's needs. By the end of the disease—severe—there may be incontinence, the inability to walk, very serious confusion, loss of speech, and complete loss of all skills to engage in activities of daily living (Reisberg, Ferris, de Leon, & Crook, 1982).

A definitive diagnosis of AD is difficult; confirmation usually can be made only on autopsy. A mental status examination, such as the Folstein Mini-Mental Status Exam, can assess functional cognitive losses that are produced by the disease (Folstein, Folstein, & McHugh, 1975). This cognitive examination is composed of 10 short-answer questions that cover orientation to person, place, and time; language abilities; memory recall; and sequencing with fine motor coordination. The examination takes approximately 10 minutes and can assess the individual's stage of disease.

For a complete understanding of the person who has AD, it is important first to understand the process of aging. An examination of the developments in the field of aging since the mid-1950s allows a better understanding and treatment of individuals with AD.

PHYSIOLOGY AND THE BRAIN

Figure 1.2 clearly delineates the regions of the brain that are destroyed slowly and in which order this occurs during the progression of AD. In the first stage of the disease, the area that is affected is the entorhinal cortex, a memory-processing center that is essential for making new memories and retrieving short-term memories. This stage can last from 1 to 9 years. In the second stage, the plaques and tangles move higher in the brain over time, invading the hippocampus, the part of the brain that forms complex memories or events during the life span. This stage can last from 2 to 5 years. In the third stage, the plaques and tangles reach the top of the brain, known as the neocortex, or the "executive region," which sorts through stimuli and orchestrates all behavior. This stage can last from 1 to 3 years.

Figure 1.2 is the basis for the theoretical framework on which the following aspects of the brain can be developed: how the brain ages, AD,

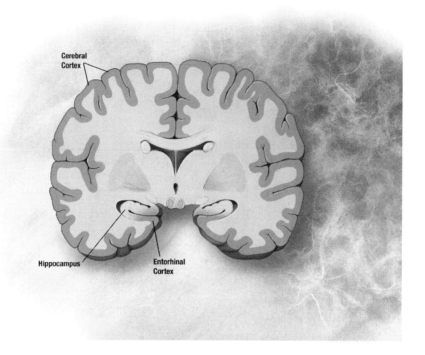

A

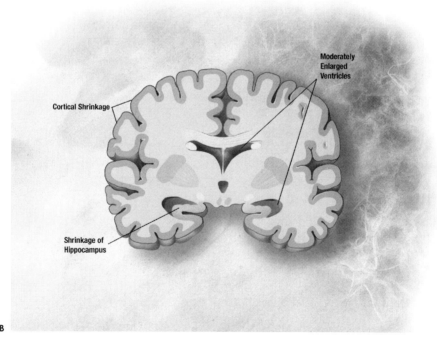

B

Figure 1.2.   Regions of the brain that are destroyed during the progression of Alzheimer's disease. *A,* preclinical AD; *B,* mild AD; (*continued, next page*).

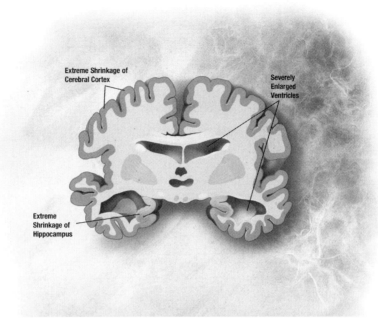

Extreme Shrinkage of
Cerebral Cortex

Severely
Enlarged
Ventricles

Extreme
Shrinkage of
Hippocampus

C

Figure 1.2 (continued). *C,* severe AD. (Images courtesy of Alzheimer's Disease Education and Referral Center, a service of the National Institute on Aging.)

and the power of therapeutic recreation. Conversation and brain activity stimulate the hippocampus, according to Diamond (1999) and Siegel (1999). This stimulation has been proved to regrow cells (Diamond, 1999). This regrowth of cells can be activated by visual, auditory, or sensory stimulation. If brain cells regenerate when brain stimulation occurs, then it is reasonable to deduce that it is possible to delay the progression of this disease from stage 1 to stage 2. This slowing could possibly delay the onset of deterioration and directly affect the quality of life of individuals with AD.

Memory and the Brain

It has been hypothesized that memory processing at the neuronal level of the hippocampus takes place only in the presence of the neurotransmitter acetylcholine. Coghill (2000) found a decrease in the amounts of acetylcholine in the temporal lobe of individuals who showed symptoms of memory loss. Therefore, with cerebral cell loss and a decrease in the amount of acetylcholine in and around the hippocampus as a result of the aging of the brain, individuals experience loss of memory and their memory functions are dramatically compromised.

According to the *Diagnostic and Statistical Manual of Mental Disorders, Fourth Edition* (American Psychiatric Association, 1994), the essential feature in the syndrome of all dementias is a significant enough loss of intellectual abilities to interfere with social or occupational functioning. The deficit is multifaceted and can involve memory, judgment, abstract thinking, thought processes, and a variety of other higher cortical functions. Changes in personality and behavior also occur.

The Latria-Nebraska Neuropsychological Battery (LNNB) was developed (Barrett, 1986) to assist therapists of various disciplines to identify the remaining skills of the individual with AD. The premise behind the LNNB is that the brain operates as a whole, yet each section seems to provide a separate function. This is an important concept that will have an impact on how the brain is understood. Many higher-level functions depend on a variety of similar skills. It has been suggested that the pathological processes of the abnormal proteins that produce the plaques and tangles of dementia progress slowly as they travel through the brain. Thus, if we can compensate for the individual's functions through areas that are still intact, we might be able to develop new systems for structural change within the brain by assessing, planning, and implementing therapeutic interventions. Therefore, the identification of the remaining skills is helpful to establishing alternative functions. Barrett (1986) addressed the significance of this new revelation regarding brain functioning in the case of dementia, noting that repetitive stimulation of already existing cell structures in the neocortex, such as repetition of previously learned behaviors (e.g., using fine motor coordination to knit or type), could facilitate memories and learned behaviors. This new understanding of how to stimulate the brain to retrieve old memories will have significant relevance in reframing the role of therapeutic activities in relationship to cognitive deterioration or early onset of Alzheimer's disease (Stern, Albert, Tang, & Tsai, 1999; Stern et al., 1994; Stern, Moeller, & Anderson, 2000).

Language and the Brain

Since the late 1990s, a trend in synthesizing concepts from neurobiology, research psychology, and cognitive science has emerged among research scientists. Siegel (1999) published *The Developing Mind,* which examined how the brain works biologically and psychologically. The following is an example of how we use language, first in a biological description and then in a social and developmental construct:

> The hippocampus and prefrontal regions mediate autobiographical memory, and thus this form of memory is directly related to an integrated spatial and temporal map. Millions of traces of perception are laid down through working memory; only a select portion will be brought into long-term memory. Of this selected set of memory traces, much fewer will survive the transition of these into permanent memory. This process of memory consolidation is fundamentally related to the biological structure of how memory is formed within the brain.
>
> A social-developmental description is the story-telling and story-listening process that often involves the essential features of social interaction and discourse. The story teller can provide verbal and nonverbal signals that

Left brain	Right brain
Speech: Using words to name, describe, define	Nonverbal imagery; minimal connection with words
Sounds: Interpret language sounds	Interpret nonlanguage sounds, music
Math: Doing arithmetic	Doing geometry
Vision: Translating letters into sounds	Recognizing faces
Tasks: Figuring things step by step, one part at a time	Putting things together to form wholes
Reading and writing	Sensing emotion and humor

Figure 1.3.   Left brain and right brain functions.

are received by the listener, and then similar forms of communication are sent back to the teller. This intrinsic dance requires that both persons have the complex capacity to read social signals, to share the concept of existence of a subjective experience of the mind.

Siegel suggested not only that memory is stimulated by the biological workings of the brain but also that the creation of narrative coherence can be facilitated by social experiences. It is by focusing on this narrative system that the important role between interactions and the brain functioning is seen: The mind is stimulated by visual, verbal, and social interactions.

Siegel (1999) suggested that the *self* at any given moment in time is filled with myriad layers of mental representations. These representations can travel through the past, present, and future. This implicit memory does not have a sense of time. It merely creates the mental experience of behavior, emotion, or perception. This is the heart of serving older adults: giving the individual the appropriate activity or therapeutic structure to share the self, which is rich with experience and wisdom.

Any older adult can utilize this "function" of memories traveling between past, present, and future because the individual without cognitive impairment enjoys the ability to reminisce and the older individual who has early stages of dementia can be cognitively stimulated by the reinforcement of long-term memories. All individuals who are still willing and able to speak, socialize, and share thoughts and ideas are increasing cognitive stimulation in the hippocampus area of the brain. Therapists, therefore, need to focus on the stimulation that takes place during a therapeutic intervention and what area of the brain is affected (see Figure 1.3).

AREAS OF THE BRAIN

Eleven different areas of the brain have been identified; each controls specific functions in the body as well as different perceptions and senses. Following is a description of each of the 11 areas (see Figure 1.4):

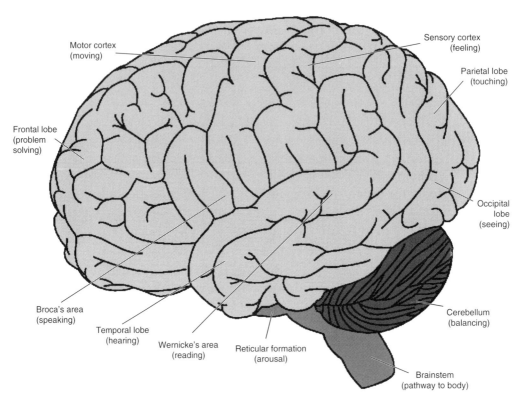

Figure 1.4. Geography of the brain.

1. The *frontal lobe* is located in the cerebrum. This region is future oriented and functions both creatively and analytically. To the right, the functions are artistic and creative. To the left is the analytical part of the mind, which deals with problem solving and complex math. The frontal lobe also plays a part in the complexity of an individual's personality.

2. The *motor cortex* governs movement and overall motor control. It is one of the primary regions in the neocortex, and many motor defects can take place within this region.

3. The *sensory cortex* involves input such as taste and smell and also is located in the neocortex. This region often is affected when brain injury or trauma has occurred; the individual often loses his or her sense of smell or taste.

4. The *parietal lobe* is located at the top of the brain. This area is associated with the sense of touch. It is the area that senses hot and cold, hard and soft, degrees of pain, and taste and smell.

5. The *occipital lobe,* located in the back of the brain, rules over vision. It discerns shapes, colors, and movements. Individuals may have varying degrees of abilities and capacities in this area.

6. The *cerebellum,* located in the back of the brain, is the center of balance for the body. It coordinates movement as it monitors impulses from nerve endings in the muscles.

7. The *brainstem,* located at the base of the brain and extending over the spinal column, is the brain path to the body. It is the center for sensory reception, and it monitors vital bodily functions such as heartbeat, breathing, and digestion.

8. The *reticular formation* is located between the brain stem and extends to the spinal column. It is the trigger area for arousal. Individuals are aroused differently. In some, it is triggered by food; for others, it is triggered by colors. The reticular formation acts as a chemical crossover for neurons that open and close with stimulation from sex, drugs, or food.

9. *Wernicke's area* is the center of reading in the language region of the brain, which is located in the neocortex.

10. The *temporal lobe* in the neocortex, located above and behind the ears, is the center for hearing and auditory processing. It receives auditory signals and identifies sounds by comparing them with sound patterns stored in memory. Research has revealed that an individual who has had a stroke can regain movement faster when rehabilitation involves music.

11. *Broca's area* is the center for speech in the neocortex and relates to other language areas. This region was first discovered in the 1800s by the French neurosurgeon Pierre Paul Broca.

LEARNING AND INTELLIGENCE

With all of this specific information about the functions of each region of the brain, it is hard to imagine that despite the same brain structures, every individual is different. Therapists ponder this every day as they look to the next new client or assessment. Everyone has varying levels of capabilities and intellect. The notion that humans all have different frames of mind and multiple ways of using their intellect took cognitive developmentalists such as Jean Piaget, Benjamin Bloom, and Howard Gardner 100 years to establish.

Jean Piaget

The Swiss psychologist Jean Piaget began his career in about 1920 as a researcher working in laboratories primarily with children. His interests focused on the mistakes that children would make while working on items on an intelligence test. Piaget came to believe that it was not the accuracy of the response but rather how the child's reasoning was developed. For example, it is common for a 4-year-old to think that a hammer is more like a nail than like a screwdriver; the logic in the child's reasoning is that hammers are found in the vicinity of nails, rather than that they belong in the category of tools (Huitt & Hummel, 2003).

Piaget developed over several decades a radical view of human cognition: Humans continually construct hypotheses and thereby attempt to generate knowledge; they try to figure out the nature of material objects and their relationships to one another, as well as the nature of humans. Initially, an infant makes sense through his or her reflexes, sensory perceptions, and physical actions. From age 1 to age 2, he or she develops a sensorimotor knowledge of the world—how objects exist in time and space. Then as a toddler, he or she develops interiorized actions or mental operations. The toddler learns that he or she can perform actions on the world of objects. At the same time, the toddler becomes capable of symbol use; he or she can use various images or elements—such as words and gestures—to stand for real objects. The toddler also is developing symbol systems such as language and drawing.

These developments reach a high point at age 7 or 8, when concrete operations develop. The child now is able to view systematically the world of objects, numbers, and space. According to Piaget, this is the last stage of cognitive development; the child is able to engage in logical thinking and rational thought. The child can go on to make further discoveries, but no other qualitative changes will develop in his or her thinking.

A generation of empirical researchers who have studied cognitive functioning have found that although Piaget's broad outline of development is still of interest, individual stages are achieved far more continuously and gradually than Piaget had indicated. It now is known that concrete operations can be solved by children in the preoperational years. Children who are as young as 3 years can identify numbers and classify simple objects, which were not believed to be possible by Piaget's theory.

Benjamin Bloom

In the early 1970s, Benjamin Bloom developed a new theoretical approach to how the child learns. In *Bloom's Taxonomy* (Bloom, 1956), Bloom theorized that the child engages in far greater and more complex activity with regard to learning and thinking than Piaget had asserted. Bloom's Taxonomy is an innovative approach to understanding the differences in learning. His theory was accepted across the United States in the educational system, giving rise to a new way to teach children so that they can learn better how to process new information. Bloom broke down the process of how we think into six levels of learning: knowledge, comprehension, application, analysis, synthesis, and evaluation.

Knowledge   Knowledge is the recall of previously learned material. In the early 1950s, students typically were taught using memorization of charts and tables. In Bloom's theory, knowledge is the lowest level of learning, because facts and figures are regurgitated without any real understanding of their meaning. For example, a cashier gives change from a purchase simply by following the numbers on the cash register without calculating the difference between the amount that the customer gives and the amount of the purchase.

Comprehension   Comprehension is the ability to capture the meaning of the information. The interpretation of information by explanation or summarization demonstrates that the learning process has moved beyond the simple memorization of material, according to Bloom. This can be demonstrated by changing the material from one form to another. For example, comprehension is the understanding of the translation of words and descriptions into mathematical figures (e.g., asking an individual to represent what 7/8ths of the whole is by using a pie cut up into 8 slices).

Application   Application is the ability to use learned information in separate and distinct situations. This could include using the rules, principles, and laws of one area in another. An example of this stage of learning is applying learned information and using it in a new or unique way (e.g., how can you locate the post office in an unfamiliar city?). Understanding and applying methods of problem solving is a higher level of learning than comprehension.

Analysis   Analysis is the ability to break down material into components or parts, so that its pattern is understood. This includes the identification of the parts, analysis of the relationships between parts, and understanding of structural principles. Analysis is a higher intellectual level than comprehension and involves the ability to categorize the information that one has learned. Once the information has been categorized, it then can be dissected from the whole to understand its meaning. An example would be understanding the various skills that contribute to an individual's ability to put work aside and go for a weekend vacation.

Synthesis   Synthesis is the ability to put together parts to form a new whole. This involves a unique understanding of the information and a plan of operation. Synthesis is the ability to use all that has been learned through knowledge, comprehension, application, and analysis to create a new or unique way of understanding and connecting concepts into new patterns or structures.

Evaluation   Evaluation is the ability to judge the value of the process. The judgments are objective or subjective and based on specific defined criteria, which may be internal (organization) or external (relevant to the purpose). Evaluation is the highest cognitive level because it encompasses all other levels.

Howard Gardner

After Bloom came the work of Harvard psychologist Howard Gardner in the early 1980s. Gardner's theory on learning, a culmination of his many years of research in cognitive psychology and neuropsychology, draws from Bloom and the findings from recent studies showing that the brain has multiple forms of intelligence that can be stimulated by the way in which one is taught.

During his research, Gardner would spend the mornings at a trauma and brain injury unit at Boston University Aphasic Research Center, where he focused on how the brain would malfunction as a result of an injury, and in the afternoons would go to his other laboratory at Harvard's Project Zero, where he worked closely with gifted and talented children to understand the development of human cognitive capacities. By researching brain incapacitation, Gardner discovered and documented which areas of the brain were responsible for various functions. Gardner (1997) then applied what he had learned in these two converse settings to develop the concept of *seven styles of learning,* in which he explains that everyone learns in different ways.

Table 1.1 describes the seven distinct learning styles: *linguistic learner,* or *word player; logical learner,* or *questioner; spatial learner,* or *visualizer; musical learner,* or *music lover; kinesthetic learner,* or *mover; interpersonal learner,* or *socializer;* and *intrapersonal learner,* or *individual.* TTAP structures each section of the creative arts programming around these distinct learning styles to ensure that each individual learning style is incorporated into the therapeutic environment. Many learning styles can be incorporated into one experience.

Learning and Perception Using Three Systems of the Brain   Gardner took Bloom's understanding of learning one step further by defining the brain as having three systems of learning. These systems can be applied to understanding how the brain takes in, processes, and retrieves information. Using the locations and functions of the brain, Gardner collapsed Bloom's six styles of learning into three unique systems that can be incorporated in and used as a structure and foundation for therapeutic programming.

Gardner's three systems are *affective, strategic,* and *recognition.* The affective system lies in the cortical and subcortical regions, which also is where the limbic system resides. This system is described as the seat of emotions, ranging from fear to great happiness. The strategic system is located in the interior and frontal lobes. This system involves planning, fine motor skills, speaking, and reading. The recognition system is located in the occipital, parietal, and temporal lobes. This system is responsible for identifying patterns, which can be letters and words. It also is responsible for identifying faces and voices that are familiar or unfamiliar. The three systems are summarized here.

Affective system: Cortical and subcortical lobes

- Limbic systems
- Happiness and fear
- All patterns of emotions

Table 1.1.   Gardner's seven styles of learners

Type	Likes to	Is good at	Learns best
Linguistic learner (the word player)	Read, write, tell stories	Memorizing names, places, dates, trivia	Saying and hearing, seeing and visualizing
Logical learner (the questioner)	Do experiments, figure things out, explore patterns and relationships	Math, reasoning, logic, problem solving	Categorizing, classifying, working with abstract patterning
Spatial learner (the visualizer)	Draw, build, design, daydream, look at pictures, watch movies, play with machines	Imagining things, sensing changes, puzzles, reading maps, charting	Visualizing, dreaming, using the mind's eye, working with color
Musical learner (the music lover)	Sing, hum tunes, play an instrument, respond to music	Picking up sounds, remembering melodies, noticing pitches, keeping time	Rhythm, melody, music
Kinesthetic learner (the mover)	Move around, touch and talk, use body language	Physical activities (sports, dance, acting, crafts)	Touching, moving, interacting with space, processing knowledge through body sensations
Interpersonal learner (the socializer)	Have lots of friends, talk to people, join groups	Understanding people, leading others, organizing, communication, mediating conflicts	Sharing, comparing, relating, cooperating, interviewing
Intrapersonal learner (the individual)	Work alone, pursue own interests separately	Understanding self, focusing inward, following instincts, pursuing interests	Working alone, individual projects, self-paced/having own space

From Gardner, H. (1997). *Extraordinary minds: Portraits of exceptional individuals and an examination of our extraordinariness.* New York: Basic Books.

Strategic system: Interior and frontal lobes

- Speaking and reading

- Fine motor skills, use of fingers

- Planning and the ability to mentally organize

Recognition system: Occipital, parietal, and temporal lobes

- Recognition of faces and voices

- Matching of objects with sounds

- Identification of patterns

Mental Stimulation and Thematic Programming   The research and theories of Bloom and Gardner demonstrate how the brain functions and how it stores and processes information. In addition, research has demonstrated that outward stimulation affects the physiological and biological aspects of the brain. The cells deep within the hippocampus multiply and grow from visual, verbal, kinesthetic, and tactile stimulation. The discovery of the regeneration of these brain cells has provided a new way to understand the concept of aging well. If the brain receives continual stimulation through activities that range from crossword puzzles to chess to painting to dance to music to reading, then cell growth is fostered, thereby keeping the brain connections alive, flowing, and multiplying.

Understanding the geography of the brain allows the specific regions that respond to specific stimulation to be identified and used for the implementation of specific activities. For example, the affective system, contains the limbic system which is responsible for emotions such as happiness, joy, fear, sorrow, contentment, and depression. The therapist can implement thematic programming to elicit specific emotions, which is good for the brain. The retrieval of long-term memories, which everyone has, is one of the best ways in which this is accomplished; therefore, creating thematic programming from memories of childhood, holidays, school, vacations, and so forth not only is beneficial from a participatory perspective but also is very healthful for the brain.

The primary functions of the strategic system are speaking, hearing, reading, using fine motor skills, and planning. TTAP uses graphic organizers and stimulates shared thoughts through conversation as a way to exercise directly this area of the brain. An example of combining skills controlled by the strategic system is writing out shared thoughts in a creative poetry group.

Planning and the ability to organize mentally can occur in TTAP by having the participants brainstorm what to do in the next stage of programming. One of the goals of TTAP is structuring programming to facilitate certain behaviors, with a full understanding of the impact on brain functioning.

The recognition system identifies associations, such as a picture to a word and objects to sounds, and patterns. An example of using the recognition system in theme programming is to introduce music as a way to stimulate the identification of objects. Another association that can occur through TTAP is that of representing objects through clay, plaster, and papier-mâché.

TTAP is a structured creative arts program that moves through all of the creative arts forms to link each project to a specific brain function. It also gives each individual a group experience that meets his or her learning style. Students of art therapy, therapeutic recreation, drama therapy, and so forth will learn that within a group are many different types of individuals with varying needs. The primary goal of a good therapist is to make each session adaptable to all levels of individual functioning. For example, a group in an adult day program environment could include an independent individual, a person who is recovering from a stroke, and an individual who has just received a diagnosis of AD. Each person has different strengths and weaknesses, which requires the therapist to create programming for all levels of functioning within the group. This is one of the most complex tasks for therapists, yet they rarely are trained to handle these situations. TTAP can help the therapist meet the individual needs of each person by first assessing which of Gardner's seven learning types he or she is.

CONCLUSION

The concept of TTAP is to provide a focus while incorporating each area of brain function with as many learning styles as possible. Brain research indicates that the brain can make new cells when stimulated and that the brain can be stimulated in three different areas: the affective system, the strategic system, and the recognition system. Incorporating into theme programming all of this research on and knowledge of the brain will provide a basis to facilitate learning using the basic principles of multiple intelligences while continually developing programming that utilizes all of the creative arts forms.

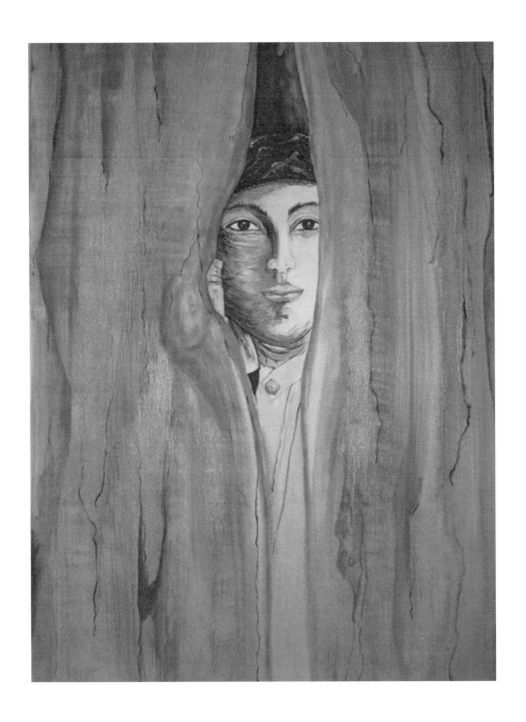

CHAPTER 2

Underpinnings of Therapeutic Thematic Arts Programming and Applications with Older Adults

Two distinct areas compose the theoretical underpinnings for the Therapeutic Thematic Arts Programming (TTAP) method: 1) theories on aging, which stress the importance of engaging in activities throughout the life span, and 2) the theoretical framework on which therapeutic recreation was founded. Developmental theory and life-span theory explain why humans do what they do. These theories also are the theoretical basis from which therapeutic recreation has grown. Having an understanding of the theoretical framework enables the therapist to create a programming structure in which to facilitate for individuals a sense of overall well-being and a sense of freedom, which leads to a sense of acceptance. From this basis, it is possible to recognize the concepts that link together to form the framework and foundations for TTAP. The theoretical framework for understanding from a humanistic perspective how humans age is derived from developmental (Erikson, 1963) and life-span (Baltes & Baltes, 1990; Baltes, Reese, & Lipsitt, 1980) theories.

DEVELOPMENTAL THEORY

Erikson (1963) provided a basis for understanding the significance of change at different times throughout the life span. He suggested that development of self is a continuous process, defined by critical periods during which aspects of a person's identity and personality emerge and change. Developmental theory is classified by Erikson into eight psychological stages:

1. Trust versus mistrust

2. Autonomy versus doubt and shame

3. Initiative versus guilt

4. Industriousness versus inferiority

5. Identity versus confusion

6. Intimacy versus isolation

7. Making a difference versus self-absorption

8. Ego integrity versus despair

According to Erikson (1982), the last psychological stage that people confront in their lives is what he called the task of achieving integrity. What he means by this is that if a person lives long enough and resolves all of the earlier tasks of adulthood—such as developing a viable identity and a close and satisfying intimacy and passing on genes and values through generations—then there is a last remaining task that is essential for a person's full development as a human being. This consists of bringing together a meaningful story about a person's past and present and reconciling with the approaching end of life. If in the later years a person looks back with puzzlement and regret, unable to accept the choices that he or she made and wishing for another chance, then despair is likely to ensue.

Self-growth is an essential ingredient in each of Erikson's psychological stages. An opportunity for this growth in older adults can occur during leisure and recreational pursuits, where significant meaning can be drawn from past experiences and used in the process of achieving integrity. "The possessor of integrity is ready to defend the dignity of self against all physical threats" (Erikson, 1963, p. 265). *Ego integrity*, as Erikson stated, is the acceptance of self in light of all other types of individuals, because "he knows that an individual is the coincidence of but one life cycle and yet all human integrity stands and falls with the one style of integrity that he partakes" (Erikson, 1963, p. 268). In other words, each individual is unique; his or her life consists of all that has been experienced and all that can be relived through memory.

Erikson (1963) specifically addressed physical deterioration in aging yet theorized that integration of ego can be mastered through cognitive processes, regardless of physical deterioration. For individuals to approach or experience integrity, they must be actively involved in society, community, and/or personal pursuits and interests that continually stimulate them. He wrote that "elders who live their lives to the fullest, participating in activities on a day-to-day basis, uncertain of or unwilling to count on the future . . . continue to behave in a fashion that takes a future for granted" (p. 58). This understanding of the human experience in the last stage of life speaks directly to the importance of being engaged in activities on a daily basis.

Erikson's (1963) concept of ego integrity includes an implied wellness of the ego that consists of a balance among emotional, social, and physical states of mind. This concept of wellness (the culmination of a sense of acceptance of oneself and a feeling of fulfillment) is embodied in three areas. First, personal fulfillment is found in the actions of the individual, in freedom of choice, and in direct action related to preferences. Second, the ability to attain wellness resides in the roles by which the individual lives and interacts with others. Third, wellness can be achieved by the individual's ability to live (by direct action in personal pursuits) with an overall feeling of individual wellness. These concepts also are the fundamental foundations and philosophy of therapeutic recreation. (Chapter 3 discusses how these concepts are interrelated and woven into TTAP.)

An important element in ego integrity is *cognitive life review*, which Erikson, Erikson, and Kivnick (1986) described as a significant mental process by which individuals, through engagement in activities, review and synthesize their entire life. Integrity and wisdom are equal and are represented as "integrity of experience, in spite of the decline of bodily and mental functions" (Erikson et al., 1986, p. 37). Therefore, engagement in activities is crucial to the overall well-being of an individual, as reminiscence is to the individual's psychological well-being. Often, therapists facilitate a reminiscence group without really understanding the significance of revisiting life experiences within a group (see Figure 2.1).

Paralleling Erikson's work, Butler (1963) incorporated the concept of ego integrity in discussing the inner process that the aging individual experiences. Butler defined ego integrity as a universal process in older people that is stimulated by aging. "Important memories and feelings are revived in order to resolve current or past conflicts" (Butler, 1963, p. 66). Both Butler and Erikson proposed that the tendency for older adults to review their past has a positive psychological, emotional, and cognitive impact on the developmental process of ego integrity and provides access to feelings of well-being.

Erikson (1963) stated that activities are fundamental elements in which the individual integrates and processes life experiences, culminating

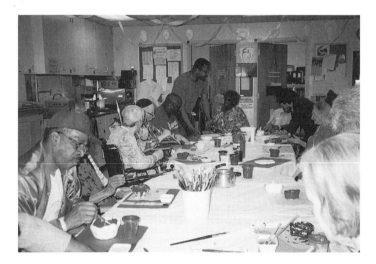

Figure 2.1. A painting program in which nursing home residents were buddied up with patients diagnosed with dementia and enjoyed painting together each week.

in a sense of acceptance of oneself and feeling of fulfillment. Erikson et al. (1986) also emphasized that promoting positive development in the last stage of life must be ensured by the individual or by the community in which the person resides: "Continued growth and development throughout old age is reinforced by either personal contributions by the individual toward their family, friends and society or by acquiring new skills and attitudes that allow feelings of personal contribution" (p. 270). Activities that are recreational, educational, or therapeutic in nature are significant to human growth and development and promote emotional, social, cognitive, and physical well-being at any age; however, they are even more significant in old age (Butler, 1963; Erikson, 1963; Erikson et al., 1986).

LIFE-SPAN THEORY

Life-span theory (Baltes et al., 1980) expands on developmental theory by viewing personal development as not only sequential, universal, unidirectional, and irreversible but also multidirectional and multidimensional (McCluskey & Reese, 1984). Change is viewed as contextual in nature and in relation to life events. Baltes et al. (1980) distinguished three types of influences on the individual—1) normative (age, grade), 2) normative historical (evolutionary), and 3) non-normative—and stated that "all three influences mediate through the developing individual, act and interact to produce life-span development" (p. 75). For clarification, *normative* was defined as a person's actual age. *Normative historical* is the individual's past, or history; and *non-normative* is the state that one is in as a result of unforeseen physical, psychological, or emotional disturbances. For example, a healthy individual is involved in an accident that renders him or her unable to walk. This person's normative age is his or her age at the time of the accident. The normative history refers to the person's lifestyle just before the accident, such as the person's job; interests; and social, community, or spiritual pursuits. The non-normative is the circumstance that the individual suddenly is living in a rehabilitation hospital and recovering.

According to Baltes's life-span theory, there is a close correlation between the individual's interests while he or she is in the rehabilitation facility and his or her interests before the accident. Participation in activities therefore is historical in nature. A person's past activity levels can predict future activity levels (Scarmeas et al., 2001). Therefore, the inclusion of history-graded (evolutionary) influences (defined as biological and environmental elements) clarifies an individual's development through his or her changing physical body coupled with a changing environment or world (see Figure 2.2).

Voelkl and Mathieu (1995) and Voelkl et al. (1996) used life-span theory as a theoretical framework to analyze the activity level of residents of skilled nursing facilities (SNFs). Residents were asked to identify in interviews and on an activity checklist the leisure activities in which they partic-

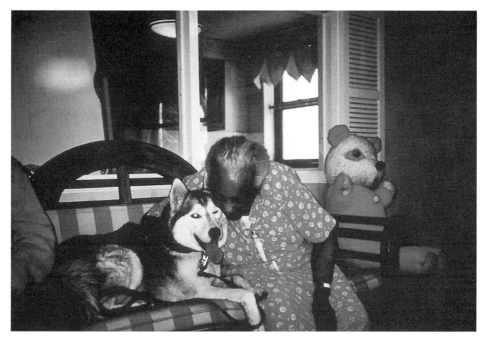

Figure 2.2.   A resident in a skilled nursing home, who had always lived with a dog, visits with a trained pet therapy dog.

ipated before and after moving to the SNF. Voelkl and Mathieu's research documented a strong statistical correlation between high levels of activity participation before entering an SNF and high levels of activity levels after moving to the SNF, which demonstrates consistency in activity participation throughout the life span. Their findings support life-span theory (Baltes et al., 1980) and demonstrate the correlation between activity level in earlier stages of life and in the last stage of life.

Life-span theory was the theoretical framework for the Nun Study (Lemonick & Park, 2001; Snowdon, 2001; described in detail in Chapter 1), which is the largest, longest (participants' ages ranged from 16 to death), and most significant research to date linking cognition, education, and recreational activities to life-span development. The behaviors (e.g., recreation activities, praying, writing, reading) of 678 nuns were followed by Snowdon since the nuns entered the convent at age 16 years. The study strongly demonstrated the relationship between activity participation and wellness. The nuns who participated more frequently in therapeutic activities were less likely to have any dementia-related illness as they grew older.

RECREATION

The field of therapeutic recreation is associated with a conceptual framework that is based on a humanistic approach that emerges from developmental and life-span theories. An understanding of what therapeutic recreation encompasses must be preceded by an understanding of what is meant by *recreation*. Kraus (1978) defined recreational activities or experiences as those that usually are chosen voluntarily by the participant either because of the pleasure or creative enrichment that is derived from them or because of a perception that personal or social value will be gained. The recreation experience, although often within a group environment, is individual and unique.

The use of recreational activities as a therapeutic adjunct to care was first introduced in facilities for people with mental disabilities in the mid-1900s. Avedon (1974) explained the development of therapeutic recreation and proposed the concept of therapeutic recreation service to prevent dysfunctions that result from a lack of recreation opportunities among special groups and to treat illness and disability.

Austin (2001) explained that "[therapeutic recreation] recognizes the importance of having the ability to be self-directed by taking action. The freedom to make independent choices based on personal preferences is essential to develop themselves through the involvement or action of therapeutic activities across the life span" (pp. 33, 149). One essential concept in therapeutic recreation is the ability of individuals to progress across a continuum of wellness when the activities are therapeutic or educational in nature or pursued on the basis of personal preference. This continuum of wellness has been described by Peterson and Gunn (1984) within the framework of health and illness: An individual, throughout the life span, can pass from wellness to illness and back again (see Figure 2.3).

According to the National Therapeutic Recreation Society, which was established in 1982, the purpose of therapeutic recreation is to facilitate the development, maintenance, and expression of an appropriate leisure lifestyle for individuals with physical, cognitive, emotional, and/or social limitations. Therapeutic recreation as part of a care plan has been researched for more than 25 years and has been shown to have a significant and positive effect on well elderly individuals and residents in assisted living centers.

In the last 15 years, researchers have additionally proven that therapeutic recreation has a positive effect on individuals diagnosed with varying stages of Alzheimer's disease and shows positive outcomes on cognition, socialization, and physical and emotional well-being in residents of SNFs who have Alzheimer's disease. Therapeutic recreation is reported to have a positive effect on cognitive functioning (Buettner, Kernan, & Carroll, 1990), improve psychosocial well-being (Voelkl & Mathieu, 1995),

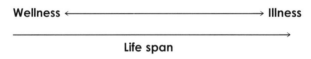

Figure 2.3.   Continuum of wellness.

(From Peterson, C.A., & Gunn, S.L. (1984). *Therapeutic recreation program design: Principles and procedures.* Englewood Cliffs, NJ: Prentice Hall.)

and improve physical functioning (Cohen-Mansfield, Werner, & Rosenthal, 1992).

Research by Levine Madori (2004) with individuals who spent 1 full year in a SNF and were diagnosed with only mild or moderate Alzheimer's disease revealed both positive and significant correlations between cognition and psychosocial well-being with increased time involved in programming and frequency in participation of varying therapeutic recreation activities. Therapeutic recreation also has been proved to have a positive psychological effect on individuals with severe Alzheimer's disease (Dunn & Wilhite, 1997; Weiss & Kronberg, 1986). Life-span theory describes a multidirectional element in relation to the importance of activities by addressing further the relationships between activities and positive physical, social, and environmental influences later in life.

According to developmental (Erikson, 1963) and life-span (Baltes et al., 1980) theories, individuals who have Alzheimer's disease and face the threat of loss of self as well as death still can attain ego integrity. Through active participation in therapeutic activities, these individuals can have positive experiences that promote emotional well-being, enhance physical capabilities, and improve overall psychosocial well-being. Concepts of therapeutic recreation that are derived from developmental and life-span theories include providing continual promotion of self-driven choices, intrinsic motivation, optimal experiences, self-actualization through freedom of self-expression, and facilitation in achieving the fullest possible growth and overall development (Austin, 2001).

Summary

Developmental theory and cognitive life review address the significance of activities in later life. Life-span theory goes further to explain that personal pursuits in society and communities foster an emotional, social, physical, and cognitive balance. Through these experiences, an individual develops a sense of self-acceptance, which fosters ego integrity. These theories also link cognitive functioning to activity participation, thereby enhancing psychosocial well-being through life experiences. Therapeutic recreation gives form and structure to organized activities, thereby enabling participants to continue to grow and develop even in the last stage of life. The largest growing group in the United States is adults who are older than 65 years. It is predicted that by 2030, 20% of the total population in the United States will be older than 65 years, and 50% will be older than 40 years. The last stage of human life now lasts longer than any other developmental stage, so the activities in which older adults participate are fundamental to overall well-being.

APPLYING THE CONCEPTS OF TTAP

TTAP is a structured way to stimulate the three areas of the brain while developing themes through which the therapeutic activity is implemented.

It focuses on a single topic while allowing the therapeutic process to unfold within the group experience. The activity process itself is important with regard to the individual's skill level and the activity challenge. When the participant's skill level is low and the activity challenge is high, the individual is likely to experience frustration and anxiety. When the participant's skill level and activity challenge are equal, however, the participant is able to achieve a state of concentration and energy expenditure that Csikszentmihalyi (1990) termed *flow*. According to Edgington et al. (1998), "For a successful leisure experience to occur, individuals must perceive themselves to have a degree of competence commensurate with the challenges of the intended leisure experience. This matching of skills and challenges is necessary for satisfying experiences" (p. 34).

Concepts of TTAP Related to Leisure Behavior

The Accountability Model of Service (Stumbo & Peterson, 2004; formerly known as the Leisure Ability Model [Peterson & Gunn, 1984]), through the three areas of functional intervention (therapy), leisure education, and recreation participation, provides specific information on service delivery content and outcomes for participants. These three areas are critical for leisure satisfaction and enjoyment. Each of these areas is reviewed according not only to its relationship to the recreation service model but also to the fundamental concepts that are promoted through TTAP.

TTAP Promotes Perceived Freedom Through Personal Choice

TTAP is based on the continual feedback given by each participant from his or her personal life experiences and the incorporation of this material by the therapist into group programming. One of the fundamental concepts of leisure behavior is perceived freedom (Iso-Ahola, 1980; Mannell & Kleiber, 1997). Perceived freedom means that the activity or behavior in which the individual participates is purely for leisure's sake (i.e., actions are chosen freely), not because someone else is forcing participation. The therapist continually solicits input from the participants through conversation and art experiences, thereby fostering participants' free will in choosing to participate and the extent to which they contribute. Because research in older adults has shown that these individuals express the continued need to participate and that participation, at whatever skill level of the individual, is crucial to well-being and quality of life (Levine Madori, 2004), the role of therapeutic recreation is to provide many opportunities for the individual to make personal choices and thereby remain a participant in therapeutic recreation activities. TTAP offers psychological benefits that include the opportunity for the participant to believe that he or she is in control of and contributing to events and activities. In addition, allowing the participant to define his or her own level of success, make choices in activities, and take responsibility for those choices are ways to individualize the therapeutic environment, thereby having a direct effect on the cognitive, emotional, physical, and social domains of all individuals, including those who have disabilities or cognitive impairment and those who are frail.

TTAP Promotes Intrinsic Motivation Through Self-Determination

Activities that are experienced successfully also provide opportunities for development of self, found through self-expression, self-development, and self-awareness. Deci (1975) and Deci and Ryan (1985) first presented the concept of intrinsic motivation as one of the essential components of the human experience. Mannell and Kleiber (1997) applied the theory of intrinsic motivation to leisure behavior and emphasized the relationship of freedom of choice to self-determination. People are intrinsically motivated by how something makes them feel. These feelings include personal enjoyment, satisfaction, and gratification. TTAP is structured around each individual in the group. Contributing to the group experience and receiving positive feedback and affirmation from not only the therapist but also other participants fosters continued feelings of gratification and personal enjoyment. TTAP relies on this constant positive outcome to strengthen the intrinsic motivation to participate.

TTAP Promotes Self-Efficacy

Self-efficacy or competence is the belief that an individual can exercise control over his or her own functions and over environmental events to reach a desired end (Bandura, 1997, 2001; Warr, 1993). Efficacy beliefs play an important role in leisure behaviors and leisure pursuits. These beliefs of competence can influence whether the individual thinks optimistically or pessimistically, thereby affecting self-enhancing or self-hindering thoughts and behaviors. Stumbo and Peterson stated that

> Efficacy beliefs are fundamental to the individual's sense of competence and control. Individuals with higher self-efficacy believe their choices and actions will affect the outcome of a situation; those with lower self-efficacy believe their choices and actions have little relationship to the outcome." (2004, p. 21).

Bandura (1997) explained that information sources for self-efficacy include 1) vicarious experience (i.e., observing someone else perform a similar task), 2) performance accomplishments (i.e., succeeding at the same or a similar task), 3) verbal persuasion (e.g., "you are able to do this task"), and 4) physiological arousal (i.e., the physical body is ready to perform). TTAP allows the participant to watch as other group members share ideas, interests, and feelings and also offers verbal persuasion not only from the therapist but also—and most important—from peers.

TTAP Promotes Optimal Experience

Csikszentmihalyi (1990) popularized the concept of being in the optimal experience as *flow*. For a person to get into the flow, a number of elements need to be present (Csikszentmihalyi, 1990; Edgington et al., 1998; Heywood, 1978; Mannell & Kleiber, 1997):

- Intense involvement
- Clarity of goals and feedback
- Deep concentration
- Transcendence of self
- Lack of self-consciousness
- Loss of time
- Intrinsic rewarding experience
- A balance between challenge and skill

Csikszentmihalyi (1990) summed up the importance of these perceptions: "In the long run optimal experiences add up to a sense of mastery—or perhaps better, a sense of *participation* in determining the content of life—that comes close to what is usually meant by happiness as anything else we can conceivably imagine" (p. 4). The optimal experience contributes to the emotional, psychological, social, and physical wellness of the individual. TTAP offers these elements in the structure of a theme program. By giving the participant the opportunity to revisit a theme continually, the art experience can be extremely rewarding and ultimately reinforce the flow throughout the experience.

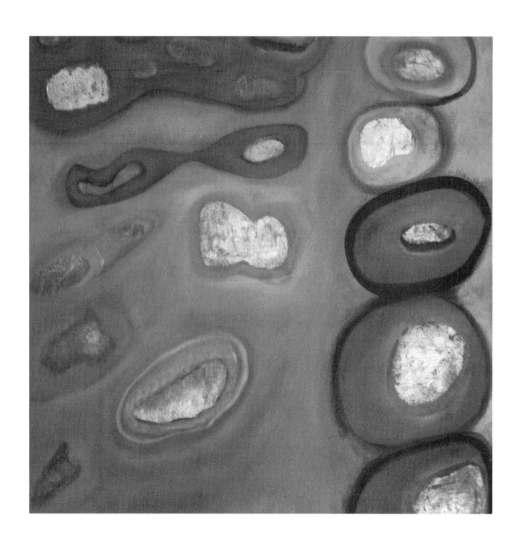

CHAPTER 3

Therapeutic Thematic Arts Programming in Therapeutic Recreation

Recreation therapists, also referred to as therapeutic recreation specialists, provide wellness services and recreational activities to individuals with disabilities or illnesses as well as to older adults. Using a variety of techniques, including arts and crafts, animals, sports, games, dance and movement, drama, music, and community outings, therapists address and maintain the emotional, social, cognitive, and physical well-being of their clients. Therapists can help to reduce depression, stress, and anxiety; recover basic motor functioning and reasoning abilities; build confidence; and promote socialization so that their clients can enjoy greater independence, as well as reduce or eliminate the effects of their illness or disability. In addition, therapists help to integrate people with disabilities into the community by teaching them how to use community resources and recreational activities.

In acute health care environments, such as hospitals and rehabilitation centers, recreation therapists rehabilitate individuals with specific health conditions, usually in conjunction or collaboration with physicians, nurses, doctors, social workers, and physical or occupational therapists. In long-term and residential care facilities, recreation therapists use leisure activities, especially structured group programs, to improve and maintain their clients' general health and well-being. They also can provide interventions to prevent the client from further medical problems and complications related to his or her current illness or disability.

Recreation therapists relate with clients on the basis of information that they obtain from medical records, observation, medical staff, family members, and personal accounts. They then develop and implement therapeutic interventions that are consistent with clients' needs and interests. For example, a client who is bedridden will be encouraged to try bedside painting or drawing; a right-handed person with paralysis on the right side may be instructed in how to adapt to using his or her unaffected and nondominant left side to throw a ball. In addition, since the early 1990s, recreation therapists have been incorporating into their programming relaxation techniques to reduce stress and tension, stretching and limbering exercises for proper body mechanics during recreation activities, pacing and energy conservation techniques, and individual as well as team activities.

Community-based recreation therapists may work in park and recreation departments, in inclusive education programs for school districts, or with older adults and people with disabilities. Included in the last group are programs and facilities such as assisted living, adult day programming, and substance abuse rehabilitation centers. In these programs, therapists use interventions to develop specific skills while providing opportunities for exercise and mental stimulation through cognitive exercises, creativity, and fun.

According to the U.S. Department of Labor, Bureau of Labor Statistics (2006), in 2002 there were 27,000 jobs held by recreation therapists. In 2005, this number grew to more than 37,000. Approximately one third of these salaried jobs are in geriatric settings, including community programs for older adults, nursing facilities, and assisted living environments; one third are in hospitals; and the remaining therapists work primarily in mental health, substance abuse, individual and family services, federal government agencies, and outpatient facilities.

The Bureau of Labor Statistics predicts that overall employment of recreation therapists will grow rapidly in the area of older adult care into the year 2012. Fast employment growth also is expected in residential and outpatient facilities that serve people with disabilities, older adults, and older adults with mental disabilities. This sequence of rapid job growth is due in large part to the growing numbers of older adults across the United States as well as advances in health care. Modern technology, advances in medicine, and overall health care are allowing people to live much longer than ever before. By 2050, it is expected that the number of adults who are older than 65 years will be greater than the entire population of the United States was in 1900.

HISTORY OF THERAPEUTIC RECREATION

Therapeutic recreation was started by three professional organizations: the hospital section of the American Recreation Society in 1948; the recreation therapy section of the American Association for Health, Physical Education and Recreation in 1952; and the National Association of Recreation Therapists in 1953.

The National Therapeutic Recreation Society (NTRS) was established in 1982 and adopted the Accountability Model of Service (Stumbo & Peterson, 2004; formerly known as the Leisure Ability Model) concept as its official philosophical viewpoint. The purpose of therapeutic recreation, according to the NTRS, is to "facilitate the development, maintenance, and expression of an appropriate leisure lifestyle for individuals with physical, mental, emotional and/or social limitations" (NTRS, 1982, p. 1). The NTRS position asserts that all humans have needs for and rights to recreation. The approach of a therapeutic recreation program depends on the level of functioning of each client. Each program requires a certified specialist to assess, plan, implement, and evaluate an individualized therapeutic approach.

Peterson and Gunn (1984), using the Leisure Ability Model, which incorporates treatment, leisure education, and independent leisure participation, developed a therapeutic recreation service model that was based on a continuum of services. They developed a tripartite theory, essentially a spectrum approach, whereby therapeutic treatment and the more clinical aspect are at one end, leisure counseling and leisure education are in the middle, and adaptable and independent recreation are at the other end. The model is based on the wellness continuum (see Figure 2.3).

Three specific areas of professional services—functional intervention, leisure education, and recreation—are used to provide this comprehensive leisure ability approach toward enabling appropriate leisure lifestyles. These three areas have unique purposes in relation to client need, yet each area uses the same delivery processes: assessment or identification of client need, development of a related program strategy, and monitoring and evaluation of client outcomes.

Functional Intervention (Therapy)

In the service area of functional intervention, the therapeutic recreation specialist creates an environment that balances between activity for activity's sake and activity for therapeutic recreation. The quality of the client's experience is important to the recreation (Weiss & Kronberg, 1986). Mobily (1985) categorized the conditions of recreation as a therapeutic treatment and identified three essential components: the therapeutic recreation environment, the therapeutic recreation specialist, and the therapeutic recreation activities.

Therapeutic Recreation Environment   In the analysis of the therapeutic recreation environment, Mobily (1985) cited the research of Langer and Roden (1976) and Schultz (1976), which demonstrated that when subjects can control some aspects of their environment, psychological benefits will result. Thus, by altering a person's perception of personal control, therapeutic recreation can produce positive changes in the psychological outlook (Mobily, 1985).

Therapeutic Recreation Specialist   The therapeutic recreation environment becomes therapeutic only when the client is given the opportunity to feel that he or she is in control of and contributing to events and activities. The therapeutic recreation specialist can individualize the therapeutic environment by helping the client find his or her own level of success, allowing choices in activities, and letting the client take responsibility for those choices.

The behaviors of the client and the specialist in therapeutic recreation also contribute to the therapeutic element of the environment. Providing a safe place where the client can receive positive verbal and nonverbal feedback helps to facilitate therapeutic interaction. The client should be made to feel, by the therapist, that he or she is responsible for an outcome and therefore directly affected by the therapeutic environment.

Therapeutic Recreation Activities   Mobily (1985) suggested that the activities that are provided in therapeutic recreation are provided for the express purpose of directly achieving outcomes. He continued that the relief of excess stress should be an aspect of the activity, thereby making thc cvcnt therapeutic.

Recreation is therapeutic when it is a directed as well as a purposeful intervention for a person's behavior. The environment that the specialist provides allows this functional intervention through recreation to take place. Therapeutic recreation services use a planned approach of assessments, written goals and objectives, implementation of functional intervention, and evaluation of an individual's progress. Therapeutic recreation is treatment oriented and directly affects an individual's cognitive, emotional, physical, and social domains.

Leisure Education

The purpose of the leisure education service area is to provide opportunities for the acquisition of skills, knowledge, and attitudes related to leisure involvement. For some clients, acquiring leisure skills, knowledge, and attitudes is a priority. The majority of clients in residential, treatment, and community environments need more leisure education services to initiate and engage in leisure experiences. It is the absence of leisure learning opportunities and socialization that blocks or inhibits these individuals from participation in leisure experiences. Leisure education services are used to provide a client with leisure skills, enhance a client's attitudes concerning the value and the importance of leisure, and to teach a client about opportunities and resources for leisure involvement.

Therapists who work with older adults often find that their clients did not attend college, and it is estimated that 40% of those who were born in the 1930s did not complete high school. Most older adults currently living in the early 2000s grew up during the Depression era, when the education system did not provide the arts, sports, and music programming that is found more commonly in the public school system in the early 2000s. Leisure education services introduce older adults to painting, drawing, tiling, sculpting, and more that they may never have experienced. Therefore, leisure education programs provide the opportunity for the development of leisure behaviors and skills (NTRS, 1982).

Recreation

The inclusion of independent recreation participation as an area in the therapeutic recreation service model provides opportunities that allow voluntary client involvement in recreation interests and activities. Clients are completely independent and often just need encouragement and opportunities to find self-fulfillment through self-expression and self-esteem. Once the client learns *how*, this independent recreation participation allows him or her to expand and grow at his or her own pace. Many older adults start in the leisure education area of the service model and move to independent recreation participation.

Dr. Bernath Eugene Phillips, one of the early pioneers in therapeutic recreation, stated,

> Can we agree—that a person needs recreation whether or not he is in the hospital. . .that he needs recreation as he needs food, exercise, rest, family, and shelter. . .that those deficient in recreation, whether in account or kind, must be prescribed recreation just as those deficient in certain nutrients must be prescribed diets. . . that further, there are many in the hospital with no recreation deficiency who nonetheless need recreation just as there are those with no diet deficiency who must eat. (Phillips, 1956, p. 52)

THERAPEUTIC THEMATIC ARTS PROGRAMMING ENHANCES THERAPEUTIC RECREATION

The three service areas of therapeutic recreation—functional intervention, leisure education, and leisure participation—represent a core continuum of care that allows individualized programming through the provision of special recreation participation opportunities. Thematic programming uses the comprehensive leisure ability approach to guarantee each individual with vastly different needs the opportunity to have control of and input into the development of his or her own therapeutic recreation programming. This level of control ensures opportunities for continued self-growth through the creative arts. This is the goal of Therapeutic Thematic Arts Programming (TTAP): allowing clients to give direction so that they may be more involved in the creation and *flow* of the therapeutic programming rather than passive consumers of activities.

All people, including those with disabilities or illnesses, have a right to and a need for leisure involvement as an aspect of the human experience (Auerbach & Benezra, 1988; Brasile et al., 1997; Broach, Groff, Dattilo, Yaffe, & Gast, 1997–1998; Caldwell, Dattilo, & Kleiber, 1994–1995; Dattilo, 2000; Dattilo & Hoge, 1994–1995; DeMong, 1997; Gulick, 1997; Nation, Benshoff, & Malkin, 1996; Skalko, 1990). The purpose of therapeutic recreation services is to facilitate the development, maintenance, and expression of an appropriate lifestyle for individuals with limitations through the provision of functional intervention, leisure education, and recreation participation (NTRS, 1982).

Mobily (1985) stated that activities in therapeutic recreation must provide opportunities that achieve direct outcomes. Therefore, if recreation is to be therapeutic, then it must be a purposeful intervention into a person's behavior so that an individual's goal may be achieved. TTAP enhances a therapist's ability to create goals and objectives that will facilitate direct and individual responses that are based on personal experiences. Allowing clients full control by structuring the group specifically toward individualized participation in the subject matter is an effective way to provide programming that has a direct impact on individuals' positive recall.

TTAP creates a creative and enriching environment that stimulates and increases the opportunities for voluntary participation. Through individual participant in a group experience, an individual can derive personal benefits because of perceived personal or social values to be gained from the involvement. As Shivers and Fait (1975) noted, therapeutic activities are a significant part of the functional intervention process. When programming is focused and developed specifically for each individual, each participant is able to personalize his or her interpretation, which adds directly to the quality of life. Often in a group, a few individuals will emerge as the "vocal" ones, which sometimes affects the ability for others to participate. The first step in TTAP, which uses structured organizational thinking patterns on a board (e.g., chalkboard), allows all to participate and none to dominate. TTAP can be adapted to all activities that are designed to sustain the health of a variety of individuals. The challenge for therapists is to provide adaptive programming to fit the diverse needs of the group being served.

TTAP is a building block for the development of all activities. Having an understanding of the nine stages of thematic programming enables the therapist to provide a structured environment in which this functional intervention can take place. This structured therapeutic programming can help to facilitate a planned approach through assessments, written goals and objectives, implementation of functional intervention, and evaluation of an individual's progress.

What Is TTAP?

TTAP is a program of activities that revolve around a particular theme over an extended period and that provide a range of therapeutic benefits. These benefits come from two avenues: 1) the arts, including language and communication, music, dance, and drama, and 2) the physiological effects on the brain by the stimulation of the different regions through varying activities.

A theme provides a focus for exploring all areas of a single topic. TTAP provides the therapist the structure for the theme from which the group participants can take off in a multitude of directions using creative arts therapy. The use of this broad-based practice of thinking can further enhance the creative process and thereby facilitate many more options. The following example illustrates the possibilities.

> A group of well elderly residents of a nursing facility had just finished a meditation while listening to sounds of waves, seagulls, and people at the beach. After the therapist turned on the lights, she asked the residents to

reflect on and visualize past summer vacations and places that they had visited that brought to mind wonderful memories. From this simple directive, the group quickly started naming different cities where they had experienced summer vacations. Using visual organizational graphic representative charts, in this case on the blackboard in the art studio, the therapist wrote down in the chart the places that the participants mentioned: Cape Cod; New Jersey Shore; Santa Monica, California; Florida, and so forth. The memories were of warm summer days full of family, friends, and carefree vacations. The therapist then told the group that they were going to start a theme project about the seashore, first using music that stimulated thoughts of the sea and then painting small pictures of what each person visualized about the seashore. Then they moved into sculpting objects that they had seen or found at the beach, placed these objects into a sand box, and told a story about each one. The last section of this theme was to create a group sculpture, which was mounted in the day room and displayed with all of the residents' names. When a theme is worked optimally, it can last throughout a season (in this case, it lasted approximately 6 weeks).

As this example illustrates, a therapist can start to explore a theme through conversation and then through creative brainstorming that is directed at a particular creative art experience with one central theme. The therapist accomplishes this by starting with an organizational system. Most declarative information can be organized using one of six standard patterns and their graphic representations: descriptive, process/causation, generalization, sequence, problem solving, and concept. These graphic representations have been used throughout the United States in elementary and public school systems for organizing information in teaching since the mid-1990s.

Descriptive patterning is a formalized way of putting creative thinking onto structured formats of charting. The charts and tables described can be enlarged on a blackboard or dry-erase board, and photocopies can be distributed to the participants (see Appendix D). The participants can follow along while the therapist documents the group's input in a large and easy-to-read format. Remember that writing, thinking, speaking, and doing all stimulate the brain. This type of programming enhances brain wellness by enabling clients continually to "use it" rather than "lose it" (see Figure 3.1). The following is a detailed description of each type of organizational pattern.

1. *Descriptive patterns:* Descriptive patterns (see Figure 3.2) can be used to organize facts or characteristics about specific people, places, things, and events. This is the simplest form of graphic display. Each participant receives a copy to start working on a particular theme. If the chosen theme is holidays, for example, then each participant can write down the most significant four holidays that they remember. Then the therapist can display on the group chart the four most common among the group. There are many possibilities for how the group can proceed to pick one

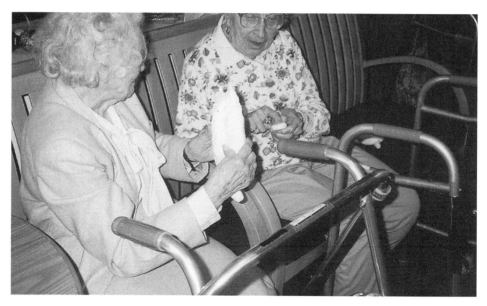

Figure 3.1. Social stimulation is essential for overall well-being. These two individuals share thoughts that are being discussed in a group program.

holiday to use as the theme. Another example of how this descriptive pattern chart can be used is by starting the group with music. The therapist can play a tape of nature sounds and then have a theme discussion regarding the sounds heard. Each individual can be asked to share a thought that came to mind while listening to the nature sounds. This enables each individual to describe a personal memory regarding a special moment or an event.

2. *Process and causation patterns:* Process and causation patterns (see Figure 3.3) can organize information into a causal network that leads to a specific outcome or into a sequence of steps that lead to a specific product, idea, or elements of a theme. If the group has chosen making flowers as a theme for an art activity, then a process/causation chart can be used to organize the many different ways in which a flower can be made. For example, a flower can be made individually, then organized into a bunch, and then placed into an arrangement. If a therapist is working with a cognitively challenged group, then this process is crucial for visually organizing thoughts and thereby preventing frustration and anxiety.

3. *Generalization patterns:* Generalization patterns (see Figure 3.4) organize information into generalized supporting information. This is a good diagram to use to back up theme information. This graphic organizer could be used to give examples of various cars that the clients owned or of types of trees that grow in various states.

4. *Sequence patterns:* Sequence patterns (see Figure 3.5) organize events in a specific chronological order. If you were discussing events in history chronologically, then this would be an excellent graphic organizer. This also is an excellent cognitive tool to stimulate recall abilities.

5. *Problem-solving patterns:* Problem-solving patterns (see Figure 3.6) organize information into an identified problem and its possible solutions. This is another excellent format for dealing with conflict or problems. It gives the user direction in the narrative, and it gives the participants the ability to interact and be heard. A good example of problem solving is when two people who live together cannot adjust to the living environment. This technique can enable clients to work out living arrangements by identifying what is personally important to each one individually.

6. *Concept patterns:* Concept patterns (see Figure 3.7) are the most general of all patterns. Like descriptive patterns, they deal with people, places, things, and events, but they represent an entire class or category and usually illustrate specific examples and defining characteristics of the concept. An example of using a concept pattern is to define a special evening event and all of the various foods needed.

Through TTAP, this visual process creates a *flow effect* while providing structure for the participants and allowing the programs to be expanded on; the typical 45-minute session can be increased to an hour and a half. Each participant works on a personal experience while supporting the group. Increased verbalization occurs naturally because the person is being asked to share thoughts that are introspective and relevant and that hold significant meaning. This flow effect will occur during each phase of a therapist's programs.

Using thematic programming, the therapist can develop and implement activities in the arts, language, and music that all link together around a particular theme. As the previous example illustrates, the group moved from a music experience to painting, then to sculpting, and finally to a group sculpture that the entire facility enjoyed. This technique can work well for the therapist who is the sole provider of recreation programs at a facility or for the therapist who is part of a therapeutic recreation department that employs several creative arts therapists.

Expressive arts therapies are a powerful healing tool. When used in traditional forms of functional intervention, these can help people release the stress that produces emotions that are known to cause immune system deficiency (Zatz & Goldstein, 1985). Expressive art also can help people maintain and maximize the body's and the mind's ability to work harmoniously with any form of prescribed treatment. It can help in the release of any negative thoughts and fears that can block the body's ability to heal physically, emotionally, and spiritually.

Graphic Organizing Tools

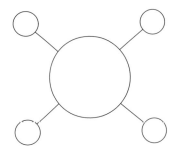

Figure 3.2.   Descriptive patterns.

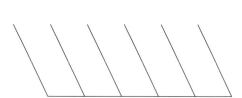

Figure 3.5.   Sequence patterns.

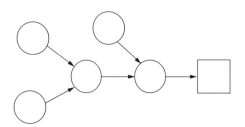

Figure 3.3.   Process and causation patterns.

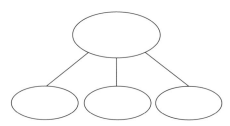

Figure 3.6.   Problem-solving patterns.

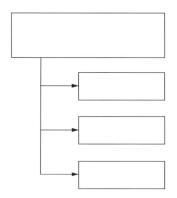

Figure 3.4.   Generalization patterns.

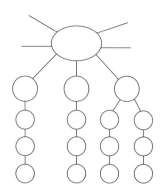

Figure 3.7.   Concept patterns.

See Appendix D for reproducible handouts.

Clinics, adult day program centers, hospitals, rehabilitation facilities, long-term care facilities, and hospices in the United States and around the world are incorporating creative arts into the practice of patient care. The most sophisticated universities and medical centers are now creating art–hospital programs that invite community artists to work with patients. The most significant factor is that it is not the product but the process that matters. Art, music, drama, poetry, and all other expressive therapies, when allowed to permeate the sterile and institutional environment in which the client lives, can open clients' hearts, minds, and spirits to the joys of self-expression and creativity.

Music as Therapy in TTAP   Music and guided imagery are excellent first steps in programming. The mind and the cells within the temporal lobe create a snapshot of emotional events, and these are deeply embedded in the sounds of music. Music activates a *flow* of stored memories across the brain; as a result, the recall of long-term memories is greatly enhanced. A good example of this phenomenon is hearing a special song on the radio. While driving to your job, picking up the kids, or running errands, you hear a song and suddenly are back in the moment when you first heard the song. That moment could have been last week or 5, 10, or 30 years ago, but all of the memories of the people, the place, and the events associated with the song are alive in your mind as if it were only yesterday. The experience of music for someone who has lived a long time is thus extremely beneficial.

Scientists as well as physicians have been intrigued by the effects that music and movement can have on the brain. Since the mid-1990s, neurological research has been finding that music and movement can be extremely useful in cases of traumatic brain injury, severe autism, profound mental retardation, and end-stage dementia, yet the effects that music has on the brain and functioning still are not fully understood. Increasingly, the benefits of music therapy in meeting the social and emotional needs of older adults as well as people with Alzheimer's disease are being researched. Bright (1988) researched music, memory, and how music and dance can stimulate memories in long-term storage, whereas stimuli such as verbal conversation can fail. Music therapy also can have a direct impact on illnesses that are associated with brain dysfunction. Consider the following vignettes that are related directly to the use of music therapy:

A client with Parkinson's disease stands in a frozen stance, unable to initiate a step forward. The music therapist starts to sing a song with a strong rhythm. The client's frozen stance is unlocked, and the client takes a step forward and then gets into the rhythm of walking.

A client with Alzheimer's disease is very confused, does not know her name, and cannot answer simple questions. She is unaware of where she is or which day it is. A familiar song is sung by the participants in the day room, and she automatically starts to sing the words to the song, along with the correct melody.

After a left hemisphere cerebrovascular accident (stroke), a client is rendered aphasic and dyslexic. He is unable to read books or magazines, yet he retains the ability to read music in complex keys fluently.

A client is in a relaxed state, listening to flute music, which she associates with a trip that she had taken to France. She recalls walking along the river and says that she can actually smell the scents of the river and the trees along the bank.

In each of these examples, the response to music is due to brain mechanisms that are involved in the perception and processing of information. Short-term memory is more rapidly eroded in the individual who has dementia, so music can stimulate memories that are still retained in long-term memory.

In clinical studies using music in association with Parkinson's disease, Selman (1988) found that music was vital in helping people with Parkinson's disease to speak. In her findings, individuals were not only able to express a larger range of emotion, but music assisted in the formation of language through sounds. This stimulation in turn allows new brain pathways to grow and connect, which has a direct impact on neurological rehabilitation.

The work of providing structures and techniques for self-expression and creativity for the aging individual is extremely significant on many different levels. The general objective of music therapy is to give all participants the opportunity for communication and socialization. Music therapy also provides the opportunity for a new means of nonverbal communication. This is especially valuable for the older participant, who may be more isolated or who may have speech limitations. Ultimately, the effectiveness of music therapy can be summarized by stressing two basic components: It stimulates emotions through dramatization while providing safety and emotional reassurance, and it opens up new communication channels. The evocative value of music is used to revive and arouse an emotional world that otherwise may be unexplored.

Words as Therapy in TTAP   Using words comes naturally but often is left out of the creative arts. In the course of growing up, people learn how to communicate tales of knowledge, experience, or bewilderment. These stories slowly but steadily become the memories that reflect a person's life. In time, stories that are in short-term memory move into deep storage in long-term memory, where they dwell in embodied silence (Rubin, 1995). The architecture of the memory system still is being discovered and still is a source of wonder. What is certain is that telling personal stories is fundamental to the human experience (Williams & Hollan, 1981); the converse, not telling personal stories, has been proved to have adverse consequences to health. Dr. Ron Kennedy (2006) states that "Nothing can be more important for your health then the unimpeded expression of emotion. Unfortunately, this is not something our culture promotes. The

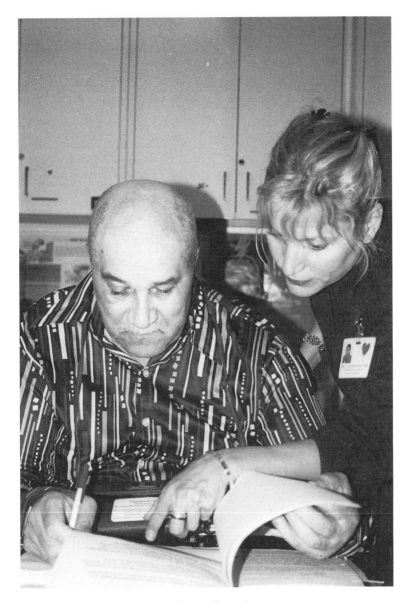

Figure 3.8. The author (LLM) assists a resident in creating a story.

result is that unexpressed emotions express their energy in the living systems of the body, frequently disrupting those systems" (Kennedy, 2006, p. 1).

Life experience and research confirm the intuitive sense that a persistent inability for one to tell his or her story to relevant people at relevant moments sooner or later becomes a problem (Donovan, 1996). Stories convey a person's knowledge and telling these stories simply is good for a person (see Figure 3.8).

The capacity to develop through learning is closely related to curiosity and can be defined as a desire to find explanation, an interpretation, or something that is of interest. Therapeutic story making, poetry, and creative writing support this vital process of constructive exploration in three ways:

1. By arousing interest and past memories in events and people that might have been forgotten

2. By providing satisfaction with explication and feedback and continuing the exploratory process

3. By providing ways to initiate, use, and develop interpersonal relationships

These are the curiosity-supporting functions that are fundamental to the use of creative writing and storytelling; therefore, writing is an essential element in the creative art experience, especially with older adults.

Photographs as Therapy in TTAP   Butler (1963) originated the concept of life review using photographs and verbal sharing to revive experiences and survey and reintegrate unresolved conflicts. Life review is the process by which a person comes to terms with the totality of the life experiences and fashions new meaning of the self. This is essential for mental health.

Weiss and Kronberg (1986) described that nursing assistants for individuals with Alzheimer's disease encourage reminiscing through old photographs. Austin (1995) described these therapeutic benefits as enhanced self-esteem, socialization, stimulated cognition, and expression of feelings.

The significant events that people commonly photograph include births of children, birthdays, weddings, holidays, vacations, and significant people and places in a person's life. Photographs elicit between people a common bond that can be verbal or nonverbal (see Figure 3.9).

Benefits of TTAP

TTAP is a structured way of incorporating and stimulating the three systems of the brain while developing and implementing therapeutic recreation activities. Programs for older adults often are the first group experience that these individuals have ever had.

The recent scientific understanding of the areas of the brain reveals how each part of the brain functions within the whole. As discussed in Chapter 1, Gardner developed the concept that people learn best when they incorporate all three systems—affective, strategic, and learning—into how they approach everything in life. Bloom's seven styles of learning address clearly how each person learns differently and are the foundation on which theme programming is built. TTAP will include each learning style:

Linguistic learner (the word player)

Logical learner (the questioner)

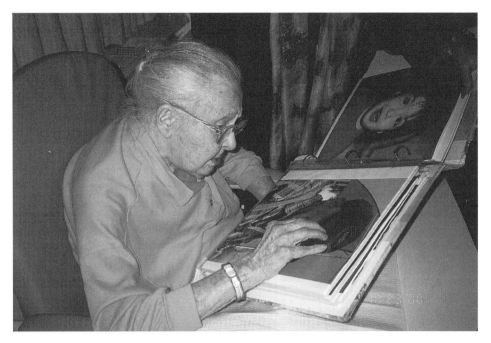

Figure 3.9. A resident is stimulated visually and verbally through the use of photographs.

Spatial learner (the visualizer)

Musical learner (the music lover)

Kinesthetic learner (the mover)

Interpersonal learner (the socializer)

Intrapersonal learner (the individual)

TTAP has a dual focus: 1) to provide opportunities for all seven styles of learning and 2) to stimulate simultaneously all areas of the brain. By incorporating each area of the brain's functioning—both right and left hemispheres—programming provides participants with continual brain stimulation. Recent research on the brain has revealed that the brain can make new cells when stimulated. This stimulation has been termed *brain wellness* (Diamond, 1999). The brain can be stimulated in three different areas: the affective system, the strategic system, and the recognition system. The most effective programming will incorporate all of this research and knowledge and stimulate all three systems of the brain (see Figure 3.10).

Theme programming is a process that facilitates creative thinking, then brainstorming, and finally implementation. The client's input is significant; it gives the individual an opportunity within a group to express individual thinking, and it promotes interaction with others and sharing of self. This technique enhances participation, allows for individualization, and maximizes self-esteem.

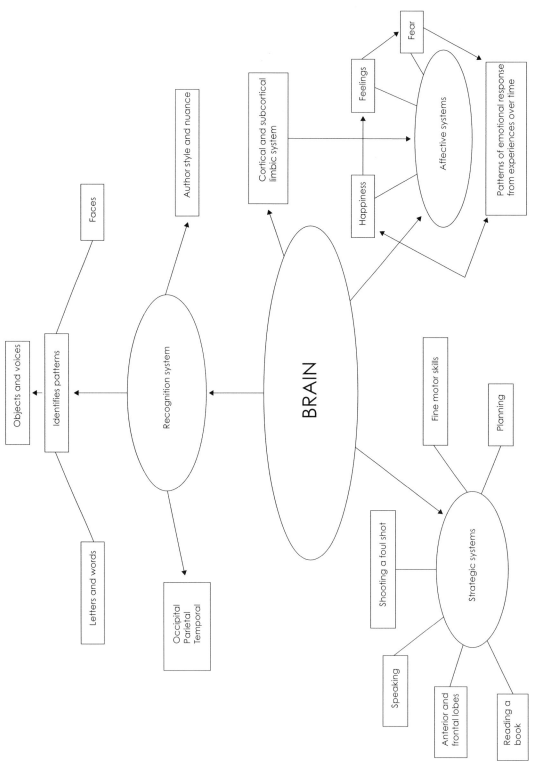

Figure 3.10. The brain can be stimulated in three different areas: the affective system, the strategic system, and the recognition system.

TTAP has benefits for the therapist as well as the participant. Often, new therapists share a similar experience: "I'm running out of ideas for keeping my clients participating." Thinking in a thematic way allows the therapist to incorporate his or her own experiences while sharing the group's ideas. It keeps the therapeutic programming innovative and fresh:

- Themes provide a natural way of learning and processing information through activities.

- Theme programming offers the participants a deep understanding of the subject or topic.

- Theme programming is structured yet flexible and is individualized to meet clients' learning needs or stimulate interests that already have been cultivated.

- Theme programming is a vehicle through which all creative arts therapies can be involved and complement the therapeutic process as well as the therapeutic outcome.

- Theme programming can establish creative activities that flow together rather than be components separate from patient care.

- Theme subjects are broad; they allow brainstorming to take place within a structured yet flexible environment.

- Themes have significant relevance to real life.

THEMES THAT HAVE BEEN DEVELOPED SUCCESSFULLY

The following themes have been developed successfully into theme programming:

changes	angels	food
symbols	life lessons	flowers
seasons	summer	family
culture	smells	jobs
systems	textures	religion
facts	fashion	holidays
communication	movies	music
languages	personalities	dances
body language	games	nations
colors	months	current events
animals	decades	women's issues
the ocean	centuries	men's issues
inventions	families	hobbies
fantasy	children	the arts
conflict	memories	the sciences
solutions	travel	the humanities
traditions	mysteries	
mountains	books	

Following are examples of how some themes have been developed. A photocopiable list of possible themes can be found in Appendix E.

Seasons

Seasons are suggested as a first theme because of their associations with everyday life. It is important to have reality orientation as part of every group; therefore, program according to the current season. First, find music that will stimulate a visual image of the season. Music can be found in popular movies and popular seasonal songs; also, check in a music store in the nature, new age, or spiritual section.

Around a visual aid such as a blackboard or a large piece of paper, have participants form a circle; ask them what the spring season, for example, means to them. In this process, the linguistic learner (the word player) can participate by using words to describe associated thoughts about the season.

After the group has offered a number of different suggestions, such as regrowth, blossoms, flowers, and warm weather, have the participants close their eyes, and introduce the music that you have picked out for them. In this session, the spatial learner (the visualizer) is able to interact with the music and visual imagery to connect to the group. This group session also allows the musical learner (the music lover) to participate by integrating music as the central focus.

After the meditation to theme music, participants again are asked to share verbally their mental images or thoughts. The therapist can use the visual aid board again to focus on the theme. The therapist's goal is to gather all of the images, memories, and thoughts into a group project. If, for example, the group collectively had many memories of flowers and gardens, then the next step might be for the therapist to direct the group to create painted landscapes from watercolors, water-soluble markers, colored pencils, or paints.

The next session could move from two-dimensional paintings or pictures to creating three-dimensional flowers. The therapist could give the group flexible wire and papier-mâché to create a floral sculpture. Each participant can create his or her own floral sculpture, or participants can work together to create a large group garden. In this session, the kinesthetic learner (the mover) can embrace the three-dimensional quality of this project.

After the large group project is finished, the next session could go back to using paper. Give participants a pen and paper and instruct them to write down words that come to mind as they view the floral group sculpture. Place these words on the large board to use as a visual aid to create words that rhyme and work toward completing a group poem or individual poems. In this session, the interpersonal learner (the socializer) and the intrapersonal learner (the individual) are able to flourish because both strengths are incorporated into the group. The individuals are asked to share, and the group socializes while doing so. This theme can progress to a special event or a photographic session.

Culture

Culture is a great theme for programs that are multicultural, because it can bring the group together by accentuating differences. Again, start with the visual aid using a blackboard or a large piece of paper. Have participants name as many cultures as they can. This will stimulate each person to share his or her own family's origins.

After the group shares cultural origins, the therapist can play music that reflects each group member's interest. The music can serve not only as a mental visualization but also as background music during each project.

After the music session, move on to a paper project. Culture as a theme has infinite possibilities. One possibility is to ask participants to draw masks on paper using cultural colors. These mask drawings then can be used to create a three-dimensional mask.

Paper masks can be purchased from many arts and crafts stores. These masks are lightweight and can be painted on using acrylic paints and glued onto, and poems can be affixed to them.

After the sculpture session, ask the group to participate in a session to create poems that reflect cultural differences and similarities; poems can be group or individual projects. As in the example of seasons, this theme can progress into a special event, such as a special dinner that serves foods from the participants' cultures.

Hobbies: Past, Current, or Future

The following example, taken from a theme program that was used in a veterans' home for men, illustrates how TTAP incorporates the various learning styles into therapeutic programming. The theme is "men's toys," or cars, boats, and trains.

In the first session, using organizational graphic displays, the therapist facilitates group discussion by starting a conversation about cars, boats, and trains and how they have changed and developed over the years. The graphic organizer can be used to structure the different cars by decade, starting with the 1920s. This first experience enables individuals with a variety of learning styles to participate. The linguistic learner, or word player, is addressed with the use of words as the central focus. The logical learner, or questioner, is incorporated into this type of visual process by answering and asking questions, thereby facilitating interaction. The spatial learner, or visualizer, is incorporated by the use of the graphic organizer. The interpersonal learner, or socializer, is given the opportunity to share with and then listen to others, thereby facilitating the social environment. Finally, the intrapersonal learner, or individual, participates because he or she can share his or her own information.

The next session could incorporate movies with old cars or race cars as a theme. The group could use paper, collages, and paints. In the next group program, the individuals are asked to paint or create a car (which could be real or fantasy) out of photographs of real cars. After that, the therapist moves the project from two-dimensional to three-dimensional, with participants using clay, plaster, or cardboard to make or sculpt their dream car. The theme of cars progresses through each creative art project. This could be followed in many directions; for example, the therapist could plan a special event and use as table centerpieces the cars that participants created. All of the cars that were made could be displayed in front of the paintings of each car. There is no limit to application of the projects; the therapist could create a program that continues for 6 weeks rather than 60 minutes.

CONCLUSION

The utilization of thematic programming in creative arts therapy can provide the therapist new ways to structure creative programming for different client groups. Theme programming naturally facilitates group activity. Through the development of a theme by both the therapist and participants, each style of learner is encouraged to participate in his or her own way within the group experience.

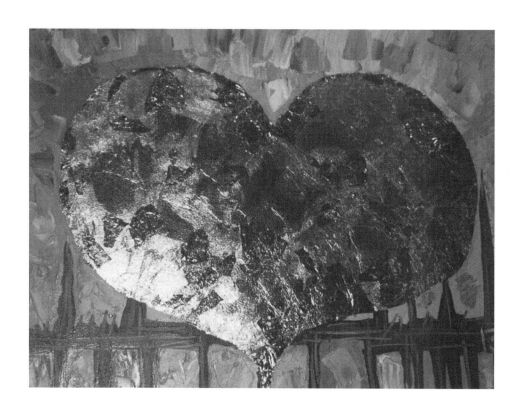

CHAPTER 4

The Nine Steps of Therapeutic Thematic Arts Programming

Therapeutic Thematic Arts Programming (TTAP) incorporates the creative arts therapies into a structured therapeutic thematic program. A significant goal of TTAP is to provide the participant with all types of creative art experiences, including writing, sculpture, movement and music, poetry, food programming, theme events, and photography.

Three main goals are woven throughout the thematic programming process:

1. Through the continual use of creativity, the therapist identifies a fundamental link among self-esteem, self-worth, and intrinsic motivation and encourages this process to take place continually within the group.

2. Through the continual use of past and present personal pursuits, life experiences, and interests that have accrued across the life span, the TTAP method elevates each individual's self-expression to a central position in all programming (see Figure 4.1).

3. Each individual's unique combination of skills, multiple intelligences, and capabilities for self-expression is incorporated.

These goals are accomplished by using connected, creative activities around a theme to provide a stimulating and rich group experience for the participants. Each individual is stimulated within the group through a series of nine steps, called the TTAP method. Once a theme has been chosen, there are nine steps to facilitate participation. The order in which they are discussed in this chapter does not need to be followed in practice; the order can be changed, and the steps can be repeated as often as the participants desire. The nine steps are as follows:

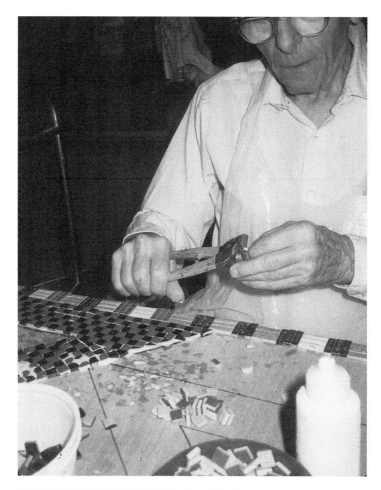

Figure 4.1.   This well elderly man is recreating an occupational experience into an art process.

Step 1: From individual thought to group ideas (linguistic)
Step 2: From ideas on the page to music off the page (musical)
Step 3: From music in the mind to the image (spatial)
Step 4: From image to sculpture (kinesthetic)
Step 5: From sculpture to movement (kinesthetic)
Step 6: From movement to words/poetry and stories (linguistic)
Step 7: From words to food for thought (linguistic)
Step 8: From thought to theme event (interpersonal)
Step 9: From event to photography (intrapersonal)

STEP 1: FROM INDIVIDUAL THOUGHT TO GROUP IDEAS (LINGUISTIC)

There are many benefits to using graphic organizers as part of the group process. Graphic organizers can be as simple as a timeline or as complex as using clusters to formulate different ideas. The following is a breakdown of six reasons for and benefits of using graphic organizers (see Figures 3.2 to 3.7) to start the group process:

1. The therapist can use a graphic organizer to illustrate and explain relationships between different issues that are discussed. The illustration and visual stimulation are enhanced by using an enlarged board to depict and define this material. The writing of the information can be designated to one of the group members, if possible, thereby stimulating the writing of words, phrases, and so forth.

2. The use of the organizer can depict information as a rewriting tool for effective lecture or information as well as demonstrations. For example, when leading a creative arts group writing session, the therapist can use the graphic organizer to focus and reflect on the topic for effective coverage of information. The therapist also can use it as a visual aid to reference. This is helpful when dealing with a topic that contains multiple components, such as how to work with clay or how to make enamel jewelry. This is ideal for clients with loss of short-term memory, stroke, dementia, or brain or traumatic injury.

3. Graphic organizers are used as a visual aid for participants who have cognitive problems, thereby ensuring visual learning while perceiving abstract ideas.

4. The therapist can use graphic organizers to assist clients who have a limited vocabulary. A multicultural aspect of group programming has resulted from the increasing amount of people who have immigrated to the United States. It is not rare to be in front of a group of clients who do not speak English as a first language or who do not speak English at all.

5. Graphic organizers can provide a visual representation of programs that will be linked through the theme. For example, the therapist might list which creative arts programs will be incorporated into the theme of traveling around the world.

6. Graphic organizers can be used to design monthly programs, bulletin boards, announcements, and various media presentations to the group, facility, or center. If the theme of spring were being used, then the monthly calendar could be designed in programming and hold more meaning to the participants.

The clients derive a direct benefit from the graphic organizer. It enhances and stimulates visual/verbal skills that often diminish as an individual ages. The need to write usually fades as a result of modern technology and telecommunications, but writing stimulates the brain and thereby stimulates cell growth.

A significant role of the graphic organizer is to organize ideas that the group is expressing and sharing; a graphic chart is used to keep a record of shared thoughts of all of the participants. If, for example, the group is for the first time using a graphic organizer, then it is beneficial for all participants to share at least one idea. This retrieval of information will help to increase participation while evoking self-esteem and self-worth. The following describes the benefits that clients derive from using graphic organizers:

1. Clients can record on their own graphic chart relationships that are being shared in the program. Just as the therapist benefits from the writing, so can the clients.

2. Clients can use a graphic organizer to organize abstract thoughts before sharing or participating in a discussion. Clients can list and organize thoughts and ideas for their inquiry.

3. Graphic organizers can be used as a prediscussion information tool. Clients can record thoughts or ideas that come to mind during a meditative session or while listening to music.

4. Graphic organizers can help clients manage their own thought process while recording how and what comes to mind first.

5. Graphic organizers can help clients prepare suggestions that they might have for presentations or display boards.

6. The most significant elements for clients are to enhance memory and writing skills, stimulate visual and auditory recognition, and continue cognitive functioning to elicit well brain functioning.

STEP 2: FROM IDEAS ON THE PAGE
TO MUSIC OFF THE PAGE (MUSICAL)

After a theme around which to create programming has been chosen, one of the six organizational patterns (discussed in Chapter 3) is selected to focus the theme and develop it into varying creative arts approaches. For instance, a simple yet effective theme to develop is seasons. Always start with the current season for continuity and validation of person, place, and time.

To begin to use music in thematic programming, introduce sounds, singing, records, tapes, and CDs that offer a connection to the theme. Using the theme of seasons, the therapist might introduce the sounds of the ocean for developing a summer theme. Once specific music has been selected, the therapist can ask the clients to listen in many ways:

1. Listen with eyes closed, blocking out all environmental stimuli; give no additional directive.

2. Listen with eyes open, sharing the experience with the group as a unit.

EXERCISE USING GUIDED IMAGERY AND MUSIC

Close your eyes and take three deep breaths. With each inhaled breath, imagine calm and cleansing air flowing into your lungs. With each inhale, visualize releasing all negative feelings and stressors from your body; imagine clean and calming air flowing into your lungs. Feel your chest and diaphragm moving up and down.

Pause.

Count to five.

1. You are becoming more aware of your body relaxing.
2. Your eyes are starting to feel heavy.
3. You are feeling more relaxed than ever.
4. You see a garden door before you.
5. Open the door and walk through the gate (garden door can be made of anything)

Listen to the sounds being heard. What images come to mind? What people do you see? What kind of feelings do you have?

Pause.

Now imagine that this garden has a beautiful forest full of old trees. You are walking in the forest, feeling completely at peace with yourself. You are exactly where you should be, right here, right now.

Pause.

I want you to imagine in your mind's eye a beautiful spot in this garden. Visualize sitting down, becoming very comfortable. Now, for the next 5 minutes (or longer, depending on the group's abilities), relax and let your mind go. Let your thoughts come and go. If you feel as though you are falling asleep, it's okay. Just relax.

Pause for allotted time, no speaking.

Now, visualize yourself getting up. Walk back through the woods. Come up on the path. Now, walk toward the garden door, take one last look at this beautiful place, your special place, to which you can always come back in the morning before you arise or at night before going to sleep.

Count backward.

5. You are starting to feel yourself.
4. You are becoming more aware of your body.
3. You are starting to feel and move your fingers.
2. Your eyes are feeling lighter.
1. Stretch and open your eyes.

3. Listen with the intent to draw out feelings, thoughts, and ideas regarding any association the person might have.

4. Listen with eyes closed and use the music as a backdrop for a guided imagery session.

This exercise can be expanded on, manipulated, changed, and/or taped to play to the group or for individual enjoyment.

Next, discuss and share what each participant experienced during the meditation. What memories were evoked; what thoughts came to mind? The next step is to use what the individuals saw, felt, or remembered in the next creative art experience. This one experience uses the sensory cortex (feeling) to remember the feelings of the meditation. The occipital lobe (seeing) is stimulated by internal visualization of the guided imagery. The reticular formation (arousal) is stimulated by the thought process and positive stimulation of endorphins in the mind and the body. The temporal lobe (hearing) is stimulated by the music as well as the voice of the therapist. While the clients share their individual insights, Broca's area (speech) is being stimulated.

The Bonny Method of Guided Imagery and Music (GIM), established in 1978, emphasizes the role of music and guided imagery in the healing process (Barrett, 1986). This therapeutic technique uses the inherent power of classical masterworks in music to evoke metaphoric levels of the psyche while uncovering feelings. Vangelis (personal communication, April 2003), a gifted musician and composer of many well-known works (the theme music to *Chariots of Fire* and *Blade Runner*), believes that the mathematical formulation of the human body is also correlated to and reflected in the music of the masters. This music in combination with guided imagery techniques creates a dream-like state that enables clients to access the vast levels of human consciousness.

The physical and emotional reactions to music can be divided into six categories: earth music, air music, fire music, water music, descent music, and ascent music.

1. *Earth music* holds deep, rich melodies and is used to explore the nature of general image exploration. Earth music also has the potential to stimulate contact with the physical level of experience, specifically within the body (e.g., Beethoven's *Symphony No. 7, Movement 2*; Vaughan Williams's *Pastoral Symphony*).

2. *Air music* has been found to be useful when traveling to the upper regions of thought and mental activity. It can be extremely helpful for problem solving and awakening the creative potential. The air sounds are flowing, free, and evocative (e.g., Bach's *Orchestral Suite No. 3 in D Major, Movement 2*; Beethoven's *Symphony No. 9, Movement 1*).

3. *Fire music* is full of energy and, more specifically, emotions. Fire music can evoke anger, passion, and struggles and awaken cour-

age through personal empowerment. Fire music quickly enables one to get in touch with strong feelings that can be hidden or derived from unfinished business. Through the experience of feeling emotions, one can express through imagery many creative solutions to problems (e.g., Bach's *Toccata and Fugue in D Minor*; Bruckner's *Symphony No. 8, Movement 2* [scherzo only]).

4. *Water music* awakens a fluid expression of feelings and connects the listener with his or her inner, subconscious world. This is a place within oneself that can hold depth and introspection. Water music helps one to give form and flow to images and enables one to feel the music and make connections to intuitive responses at deep subconscious levels (e.g., Beethoven's *String Quartet in C Major, Opus 131*; Brahms's *Symphony No. 2, Movement 3, Andante*).

5. *Descent music* can bring up feelings that may have been hidden from the conscious self. These feeling that have been pushed out of awareness must be regarded cautiously because the music has the ability to stir up many emotions, which can have an overwhelming effect on the individual. The therapist must be very careful when using this form of music. Often, as believed in Jungian psychology, when this dark place is visited, the light of salvation can be found (e.g., Beethoven's *Symphony No. 3 ''Eroica,''* *Movement 2*; Holst's *The Planets, Saturn*).

6. *Ascent music* is uplifting and expansive. It holds the power to lift emotions and thought patterns. It can evoke feelings of joy, love and happiness, and spiritual transformation. It can be used to change a mood of the group. Often, especially in the winter, therapists encounter feelings of sadness, moodiness, and sleepiness among their clients. This music can stimulate the mind and provide a feeling of refreshment (e.g., Bach's *Mass in B Minor, ''Qui Tollis''*; Mozart's *Vesperae Solennes, Laudate Dominum*).

An expanded list of music suggestions that represent the six categories of GIM is provided in Appendix C at the end of the book.

STEP 3: FROM MUSIC IN THE MIND TO THE IMAGE (SPATIAL)

One does not have to be an artist to draw (see Figure 4.2). One does not have to be an artist to draw! This statement needs to be stated and restated, so get used to it! Making art is all about the individual process, not the final product. Especially among older adults, there is a preconceived notion that one must be an ''artist'' to draw a picture. Not true! Remember, as mentioned previously, the older adults today have had little education and even less experience with making art. Even if one has never picked up a pencil, it is not too late. A client once was asked whether he had ever

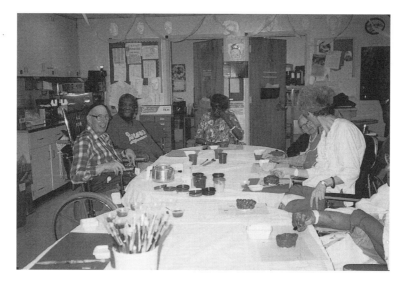

Figure 4.2.   Individuals are seen here enjoying a group painting experience.

painted. He replied, "I painted houses all my life, and I never want to paint again!" This client turned out to be an avid participate in his art groups.

Once the therapist has conducted a music and guided imagery session, each client has very clear images in his or her mind's eye. The therapist can jump from the mind to the paper by asking the clients to draw an image that they remember from the meditation. If the group is scheduled only once a day or once a week, then the therapist can refresh clients' memories by playing the music in the background. There are many ways in which to conduct this process. Most individuals are very intimidated by the pencil, so the therapist may want to start by using magazines that the clients can scan for images to cut out and glue onto paper. The therapist can give a directive to draw around the photograph so that the empty page is not an intimidation factor in the creative process.

Along with images cut from magazines and pasted onto paper, the therapist can draw part of a garden fence and then ask clients to complete the image. This works well with clients who have difficulty with fine motor coordination, such as those who have had a stroke. If the client has total loss of the dominant hand functions, then the therapist can cut photos out of magazines to assist the client in making a collage of the theme.

When a therapist is working with a group that is cognitively unimpaired, he or she can have a conversation session about the artwork. This sharing of feelings and thoughts must be done in utmost confidence, and it is recommended that the therapist say so before starting the exercise. The clients also should be asked whether they are open to sharing; there might be someone who does not want to share. Always honor the individual's feelings about his or her work.

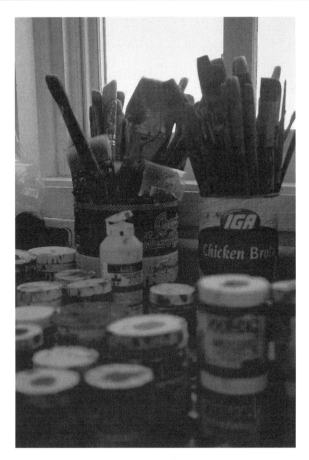

Art supplies.

Processing Artwork with Your Clients

The following questions can be helpful for stimulating and motivating the group to verbalize about their artwork after making it. The therapist's responsibility is to be a facilitator, coach, guide, or mentor, not the interpreter. The therapist's job is to be present emotionally and physically. Most successful group experiences occur when the therapist has provided a safe environment in which the participants feel comfortable to share their thoughts and inner feelings with the group and with the therapist. The following questions can aid the therapist in achieving a deeper symbolic understanding about the meaning of the artwork to the client. The therapist may want to take notes on what is shared during this type of session.

Describe your experience during the visualization. What images, if any, did you see? If this was the first time that you did guided imagery, how did you enjoy it?

How do you react to this piece of artwork now? Does it reflect what you felt or saw? Elaborate on how this artwork makes you feel.

As you look at the drawing now, what else comes to mind? Would you change anything, or did anything happen while in the process of the art that changed for you?

While doing the artwork, did any thoughts of which you had been unaware come to mind? Were there any new connections to the meditation and the artwork?

Look at the colors. Do they reflect different emotions that you felt?

Overall, how did this experience feel?

Once everyone has completed his or her work, the therapist can mount each client's work, or often the group wants to cut out parts of each person's finished work to create a group collage/mural. This technique works well when you have participants with varying abilities. Always finish any artwork with framing, matting, or mounting, and label clients' names in a professional manner. Remember, the way in which the therapist handles and displays artwork is reflected in the way that others will view and respect the work.

In this process of going from imagination to image, the frontal lobe (problem solving) is one of the active components at work. The motor cortex (moving) is needed for the fine and gross motor skills of cutting, pasting, and drawing. The parietal lobe (touching) is stimulated by the manipulation of art materials, such as feeling the paper and other materials. The occipital lobe (seeing) is stimulated by the activity in the environment. The reticular formation (arousal) is stimulated by the identification with the process of making art and self-esteem. Individuals feel good about themselves when they are participating in an activity that is meaningful. Broca's area (speech) is active as a result of the social element in the creative arts group process. Imagery is the body's and the mind's inner language; art is the voice and expression of that nonverbal language. Using art can enable the individual to connect, possibly for the first time, to an emotion or an event that has not been thought of for decades. It also can stimulate emotional healing through the connection of the deep and innermost feelings.

Expressing emotions through color, form, shape, and image releases memories. These memories can be positive, but they also can be negative. Be prepared to handle feelings of loss or sorrow that might be expressed. If an individual in the group does experience a sorrowful memory, then there are steps that the therapist can take to promote feelings of safety and comfort. First, ask the individual whether he or she would like to share what is making him or her feel emotional. If the individual wants to talk with the group, then promote the sharing. If the individual does not want to talk, then make sure that he or she is not left alone. Have a nurse, friend, or staff member comfort him or her in private. Often, people cry to express feelings of sorrow over a loved one. The following happened during a large (300-person) group meditation:

After the guided imagery, the lights were turned on and a woman was crying in the center of the room. The therapist approached her and asked whether she could share what had happened. She said that she needed a few minutes to get herself together, and a close friend who was with her took her out of the room. After approximately 10 minutes, she returned and raised her hand. The therapist was discussing with the participants the feelings and visualizations that they had had during the meditation. The therapist addressed the woman, and the woman told the audience that she had a vision of her deceased father during her meditation and he came up to her and gave her a hug and told her that he loved her. She shared with the group that her father had been a cold man and did not ever hug his daughter ''and never while he was alive'' said those words. She was crying from happiness because, as she explained, the meditation was so real that she believed that it was his way of coming to her and letting her know just how much he had loved her.

STEP 4: FROM IMAGE TO SCULPTURE (KINESTHETIC)

Once the group has completed work with paper and paints, encourage clients to share with the group what they have created. Sharing feelings, experiences, memories, and creations is an integral component of the group process in TTAP. Some people will be more willing to share than others. One way to encourage sharing is to change the physical seating arrangement. If clients are at individual desks, then rearrange the chairs to prompt sitting in a circle. The circle represents the group, and every member of the group makes up and completes the circle.

Always allow clients to opt out of sharing their work if they choose. Respecting the individual's needs is extremely important to the process of making art, expressing oneself, and fostering self-esteem. Remember that each individual is taking something deep inside of him- or herself and putting it ''out there'' for everyone to see. This can be extremely difficult for some people, yet with continual positive feedback from the therapist, trust develops between the individual and the therapist as well as between the individual and the group (see Figure 4.4).

As each person shares his or her artwork, the therapist should look for common elements and images that are emerging. These common images will help the therapist move the group to the next phase: the development of a three-dimensional sculpture from the two-dimensional format (see Figure 4.3).

The therapist focuses conversation on the common elements and continually encourages conversation within the group. The therapist's role is to listen, possibly record, but always to try to synthesize creatively the images and information given to reach the next level. Asking questions of the group is effective. Open-ended questions that do not elicit a yes or no response are ideal to encourage conversation. As the therapist looks around at everyone's work, he or she should take notice of what they have in

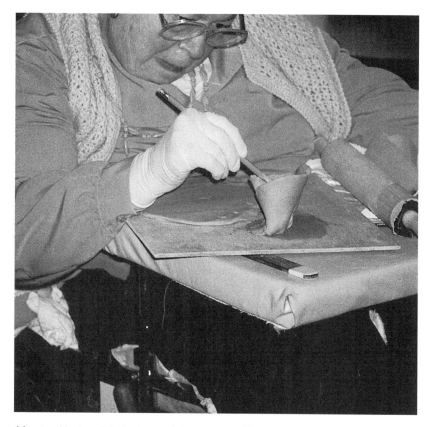

Figure 4.3.   A resident participates in a sculpture program. Fine motor coordination, cognitive concentration, and overall enjoyment are evidenced.

common. Are there common colors that have been used by everyone? What are common elements among the artwork (e.g., are airplanes in every picture)? Use these commonalities to move to another theme within the group. The theme that emerges will facilitate the sculpture project. (When dealing with a large group, the use of a blackboard or flipchart to list suggestions is a helpful tool for the therapist.) Following is an example of this process:

> *Clients with mild Alzheimer's disease had created animal sculptures from a beach visualization. The sculptures were placed on the carpeted floor in front of the participants and the group started to relate their individual sculptures to the surrounding sculptures. For instance, one man said, "Place the turtle swimming after the fish," and another participant said, "Place the large fish swimming after the smaller ones," and so forth. From this session, the idea arose to place the clients' sculptures in plaster and cover them with sand. The free-standing sculpture then was displayed in the facility with all of the participants' names (see Figure 4.4).*

Family members enjoy the verbal and visual opportunities that mounted

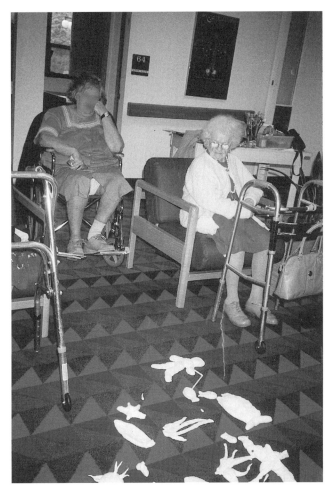

Figure 4.4. In a conversation group after a sculpture program, residents share the sculptures they made and speak about the interrelationship of one to another.

art affords them. These conversations with family members about the artwork allow the participant to feel a great sense of accomplishment and pride.

Occasionally, the group may not be able to come up with any ideas. The therapist must be creative enough to brainstorm with the group and offer insight and direction when needed. Following is an example of how to handle this problem:

The theme was summer, and everyone happened to draw pictures with balloons. As a group, they could not come up with a sculpture idea. After thinking about it for a while, the therapist decided to use balloons as the basis of a sculpture. At the next session, the therapist discussed her thought process with the group. Everyone was excited at the idea of covering a blown-up balloon with Rigid Wrap (see Appendix C). After the balloons hardened, the therapist used a sharp knife to cut the round, hollow shape into two parts, revealing the inside layered patterns. The clients then were given colored feathers and paints to decorate their egg-like shapes. Last, these shapes were glued, using a hot-glue gun, onto hard 1/4-inch foam board in a pattern that was designed by the group (see Figure 4.5).

This experience used the sensory cortex (feeling) in the sensations from the sculpture and the materials used. The occipital lobe (seeing) was stimulated by the external visualization of the process. The reticular formation (arousal) was stimulated by the thought process and positive stimulation of endorphins in the mind and the body. The temporal lobe (hearing) was stimulated by the group's ongoing conversations as well as the voice of the therapist, and while the clients shared their individual insights, Broca's area (speech) was being stimulated.

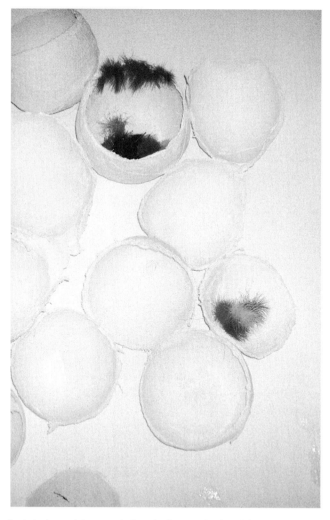

Figure 4.5.   The final plaster sculpture made from ballons and colored feathers.

STEP 5: FROM SCULPTURE TO MOVEMENT (KINESTHETIC)

Now that four steps of TTAP have been completed successfully and many opportunities for cognitive, emotional, physical, and social interactions have been provided, movement to music programming can provide the opportunities for the clients to explore their bodies in space, using directives accompanied by music. Movement also enables each individual to share common feelings, share common emotions, and express feelings in a relaxed and safe group experience (see Figure 4.6).

In the last stage, the group created some form of sculpture; in this stage, that form is transformed into something that can be used as a prop around which to move. For example, a balloon plaster sculpture was made in the last segment; continuing to use the balloon theme the group can use balloons to toss around to varying forms of music. The object, or prop, moves the individual's focus of self into a nonthreatening position that

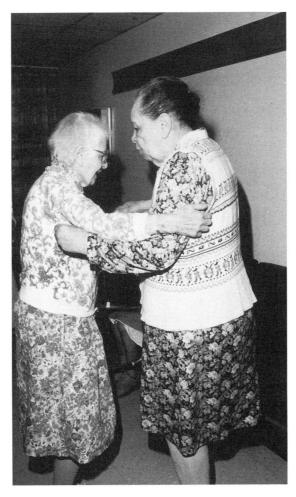

Figure 4.6. Two women enjoy a dance and movement program.

projects the interest onto the object. Movement occurs with minimal self-consciousness. Many older adults lack physical activity in their daily lives, even going for walks. When individuals live in retirement apartments, elder homes, or nursing facilities, there is a need for increased movement programming.

Using Props in Movement Programs

Motivation is a continual challenge, and the use of props can motivate movement within the group experience. Following is a description of props that have been successful in beginning movement group programs. Some movements to music programs do not need props. Many music therapists have written about the use of movement to focus on the individual's body. This technique of moving to and from the self can be explored using various body parts. Open/close, widen/narrow, expand/contract, grow/shrink, and fold/unfold are common directives that can be expanded on as well as used in conjunction with each other. If the group is being conducted for the first time, then the order should be to introduce an object first and then move into just moving the body; this is less threatening, and a greater group cohesiveness can be obtained.

Balls, Balloons, and Frisbees   Use balls, balloons, and Frisbees for warm-up exercising, alone or in conjunction with music. Objects take the individual's mind off of the body and project focus onto the object, thereby providing a feeling of security and safety. Objects also are a good way to have participants introduce themselves; they state their name while holding the object, then throw it to the next person in the group. Using the object in competition is another good warm-up; pass the object to the beat of the music, and see how long it can be tossed before falling.

Scarves   The use of scarves can stimulate and motivate the most difficult groups. The movement of fabric is a good point of departure to moving into body movements. Long pieces of fabric can be obtained from a fabric store as remnants and are not costly. These colorful pieces of fabric lower the participants' resistance so that they can be directed to move different parts of the body. Fabrics also work well when orchestrating the group to move together as a whole to form a cohesive group experience.

Musical Instruments   The therapist can use musical instruments to introduce music that has different beats. Instrumental use also is a good way to find each person's personality within the group. This can be achieved by having each member play his or her own rhythm or beat and have the other members of the group repeat and prolong the beat. Another directive is to have each individual add his or her own ending to the last person's beat, thereby creating an entirely new musical rhythm.

Audiotapes and CDs   There are so many cultural movies and musical tapes on the market that can be used as a tool in movement and music programming. Additionally, musical CDs of nature sounds, African drumming, and Brazilian music can be utilized in movement groups and then be used in discussion sessions. Look to purchase audiotapes and CDs that can be creative departures from just making sounds.

Common Exercise Equipment   Many different exercise products can be used in music and movement programming. Weighted balls, elastic bands, and weight belts for feet and arms all can be used in group work.

Categories of Music Therapy Programming

In the work of Nordoff and Robbins (1977), music therapy programming can be divided into six categories.

Listening and Choosing   In listening and choosing, the therapist introduces musical instruments that have been bought or made. These can include cymbals, harp, xylophone, drums, or any other musical or rhythmic instrument. Clients then choose which one they would like to explore. It is interesting to observe and document which instrument is chosen and whether the client explores different instruments over time.

Music-Making Client/Therapist   The therapist invites each participant individually to explore the instrument that was chosen and play it. The therapist can support the clients by playing the same instrument along with each client. If an individual does not want to choose, then the therapist should make a choice that is based on the individual's responses. Observe the following: the way that the individual interacts with the musical instrument, the nature and the tone of the music, the feelings that are connected to the music, and whether there is contact and involvement of the client to the therapist or to the group.

Group Observation   Observe how the group influences each participant. Does the group influence the individual in any way, either positive or negative? Does the individual have eye contact with group members? Does the individual have interactions and associations with the group members? Finally, which emotions does the client have after this experience?

Anticipating and Combining   The therapist can ask participants to imagine which instruments would work well together and sound well when played together. Observe whether the client can still use abstract thinking in this directive.

Memory and Recognition (for Clients with Cognitive Impairment)   Do the clients recognize the therapist when he or she enters the room, or do they show recognition only when the therapist speaks of music or even after the therapist brings out the instruments? Do they remember any components to a song?

Associating   Associative listening is the evocation by music or a musical excerpt of a subjective, affective reaction. Five musical excerpts, each representing a set of values, are played: 1) old age, 2) action, 3) religion, 4) childhood, and 5) warmth. After the music selection is played, the therapist asks the clients to choose from the above list which association is best. The therapist explains the process that is going to take place before actually doing the session. Discussion of what the value of the words is to each individual follows.

Music, Movement, and Now Dance!

The therapist can start the dance and movement session with discussion of what already has taken place. Remember that conversation and continual interaction increase brain functioning. The primary goals of this component of programming is to motivate movement through the fostering of self-expression. This self-expression, represented in dance format, can be very exciting for older adults because dance was one of the only "real" recreational activities that was free and socially accepted during the first part of the 20th century. Older Americans in early 2000s lived through very hard financial times; as a result, many are undereducated and did not experience leisure activities as they exist today. Following is an illustration of using dance as a theme:

> The group has been exploring the theme of cultures; they have drawn different flags and painted various masks and now are listening to different cultural music, such as African tribal drums and Caribbean steel bands. Fabrics can be used to make long skirts for the women and ties for the men. The music from a particular culture that has been incorporated into the group discussions now is played, and the participants explore dance moves and make up a dance around the colors and music of a chosen culture.

This experience stimulates the sensory cortex (feeling) through the actual feeling of objects used in the movement and dance process. The occipital lobe (seeing) is stimulated by the external visualization of the process that the participants are witnessing and implementing. The reticular formation (arousal) is stimulated by the thought process and positive stimulation of endorphins in the mind and the body. The temporal lobe (hearing) is stimulated by the music, the group's conversations, and the voice of the therapist. While the participants share their individual insights Broca's area (speech) is being stimulated.

STEP 6: FROM MOVEMENT INTO WORDS—POETRY AND STORIES (LINGUISTIC)

The group now is ready to engage in the many creative uses of words: creative writing, poetry, story making, and storytelling. For older adults in the early 2000s, computers, e-mail, and telecommunications did not exist. This is a generation of people who used the written word to communicate.

Getting Started

Moving from movement and dance into words is fun and creative. First, revisit your theme by possibly recording your movement and dance sessions or listening to the music used. To get started, hand out writing materials and then direct participants to list words that they associate with the theme. The therapist can use a blackboard while participants write in their own books or papers supplied. It is important to have notebooks, binders, or some other form of bound paper so that the participants can keep whatever they write in the same place.

After each person has created a free-flowing list of words, the participants can be asked to share their best three words with the group. The group can use these words to create a poem, story, or haiku.

1. *Creating a group poem:* This exercise is done by simply recording on a blackboard or large pad of paper all of the words shared by the group. Then, using the format of who, what, when, where, and how, fill in and create a poem that flows together and toward the theme. Another method is for each person to write one sentence and then have the group put the sentences together as one.

2. *Creating a group story:* Creating a story with older adults can be based on morals such as good and bad, right and wrong, and problems and solutions. Allow participants to express what has gone right or wrong in their lives, if they choose. For some, this may be the first time that they reconcile with the idea that some things that happened in their lives were not their fault. This type of group work again is significant for what Erikson (1982) called the task of achieving integrity. The group is a holding container (Winnicott, 1965) for each person to validate his or her wisdom, in reflection and sharing.

3. *Creating a haiku:* Haiku is a form of Japanese poetry that is very simple and easy to learn. A haiku consists of three lines: The first line contains five syllables, the second line contains seven syllables, and the third line contains five syllables. When working with cognitively alert older adults, this form of poetry allows for a successful educational atmosphere. After the individuals have made their own haiku, the group can combine them or start over to create a group poem using this format.

Life stories hold enriching tales of wisdom. Ask the group to share in writing a story or event that relates to the theme. Sharing these stories can create bonds that will continue after the therapist leaves the program, and it allows all individuals to experience themselves but also to experience themselves in others. Recognizing common responses to life's ups and downs brings people closer together. These stories are a window into the past and offer the individual another moment to relive a great experience, for themselves and for the others.

This experience stimulates the sensory cortex (feeling), in the feeling of the words and the writing materials. The occipital lobe (seeing) is stimulated by the external visualization of the story that is being written. The reticular formation (arousal) is stimulated by the thought process and positive stimulation of endorphins in the mind and the body. The temporal lobe (hearing) is stimulated by the group's ongoing conversations and the voice of the therapist. While the participants share their individual insights, Broca's area (speech) is being stimulated.

STEP 7: FROM WORDS INTO FOOD FOR THOUGHT (LINGUISTIC)

Food is a significant part of every culture. Both life and death are celebrated using specialized presentations of food. People socialize around eating while connecting emotionally to family and friends throughout the life span. Food can represent the various cultures in which people have been raised. Food represents various holidays that are celebrated (see Figure 4.7).

Food is an excellent source of creative programming. Food is an activity that truly affects all senses (taste, touch, smell, sight, and hearing) as well as the cognitive, emotional, and social domains. Food can be used in theme programming by counting; creating; mixing; cutting; distinguishing

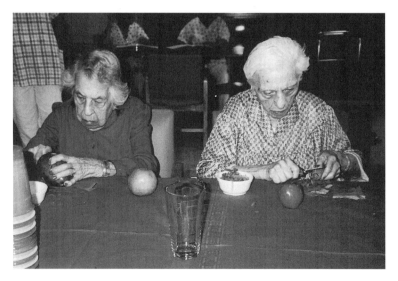

Figure 4.7. Residents cut and prepare apples for a pie.

textures; categorizing by animal, mineral, or vegetable; sorting by color or shape; and so forth.

Culture is symbolized through the different foods as well as the different preparations of the same ingredients. A room full of strangers can be brought together by talking about food, touching and feeling different foods, preparing food, and using food in innovative ways in therapeutic programming. The use of the "Food for Thought" programming came out of the work of Janet Larghi, M.S., CTRS, the author (Linda Levine Madori, Ph.D.), and the Cabrini Nursing Home in New York City. In this creative program food is used as the creative object as well as a tasty treat!

Continuing with the summer theme, ask the group to name different summer fruits; these fruits then can be used to make a salad. Have participants cut up the fruit and count the seeds. They can plant the seeds in small containers so that they can take their seeds home. Some long-term care facilities might have an area in which to grow fruits and vegetables; each week, a person can be in charge of watering, and by the end of the summer, the produce can be picked and eaten be participants in a group luncheon. Food for thought is a great way to motivate participation and enhance social interactions.

Another way to use food is to ask each individual to share a recipe with the group. More and more facilities are adding cooking as a creative component to programming. In this manner, memories are stimulated while enhancing self-esteem. Food and the preparation of food usually have been taken out of a person's daily functions when he or she enters a residential facility. The continued effort to enrich life through creative programming can be achieved by adding food. Specific foods often can trigger significant memories that have been long forgotten. Candy is a great starting point. Candy can hold early childhood memories and elicit wonderful feelings. Candy also is involved in celebrations in many cultures.

This experience stimulates the sensory cortex (feeling) in the taste and feel of the foods and the materials. The occipital lobe (seeing) is stimulated by the external visualization of the process that is involved and implemented. The reticular formation (arousal) is stimulated by the thought process and positive stimulation of endorphins in the mind and the body. The temporal lobe (hearing) is stimulated by the group's conversations and the voice of the therapist. While the participants share their individual insights and favorite foods, Broca's area (speech) is being stimulated.

STEP 8: FROM THOUGHT INTO THEME EVENT (INTERPERSONAL)

In almost every facility, adult day program center, hospital, rehabilitation center, and psychiatric unit, there are parties and celebrations of special events. Using parties to tie into theme programming is a way to display all of the group's efforts. Decorations can be made in art groups using the party theme and incorporating that theme into centerpieces. Pictures for the walls can come out of the painting programs. Table dressing, including creative napkins rings and placemats, can be incorporated into theme programming.

The food-for-thought program can organize the food and create the shopping list for the party. The group can create thematic invitations and menus for the guests. Some facilities, such as long-term care and assisted living, allow residents to prepare their own food.

The musical selection can grow out of your movement-to-music group. Hold discussions about what would be the best music for the theme. Show a movie that depicts a special time of year that is being highlighted. Individuals can create murals on windows using watercolor paints to enhance the event.

Special parties are another way to bring the community into the program. Invite family members and friends to the events to show them how the creative arts enhance the quality of life of the participants. Parties also are a good time to encourage people who might be interested in joining the group to participate.

Birthday parties, bingo evenings, Las Vegas night, and cabarets all are great themes around which to program. If the facility is having a Las Vegas night, then start the theme programming with the state of Nevada, then move to the recreation component in games, gambling, and tourism. Finally, Las Vegas–style costumes can be designed and then worn at the special event. Theme programming is a way of thinking, connecting one event to another, and enriching the lives of participants while enriching the therapeutic programming.

This party experience stimulates the sensory cortex (feeling) in the actual feeling of the environment, decorations, and the memories stimulated. The occipital lobe (seeing) is stimulated by the external visualization of the process that participants are witnessing and experiencing. The reticular formation (arousal) is stimulated by the thought process and positive stimulation of endorphins in the mind and the body. The temporal lobe (hearing) is stimulated by the activities surrounding the party. While the participants interact with each other and share their individual insights, Broca's area (speech) is being stimulated.

STEP 9: FROM EVENT INTO PHOTOGRAPHY (INTRAPERSONAL)

When working with older adults, the therapist often experiences the individuals' cognitive decline. Often, individuals need assistance in accessing memory. Photographs are a powerful way to stimulate retrieval of memories and can be used to create collages (see Figure 4.8). I once was conducting a guided imagery and art session with residents who were not impaired cognitively but were living in a nursing home. One of the group members drew a picture of a piano and when asked to share the work, she went into a detailed description of a piano that she had owned as a child and

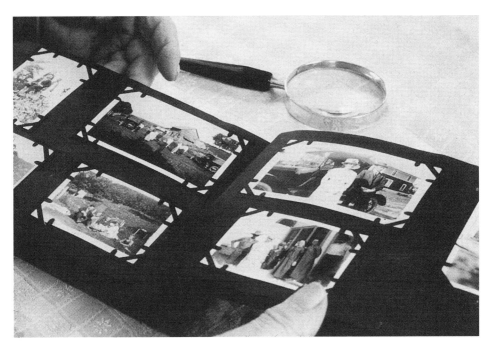

Figure 4.8. Residents work with photographs from past or present, stimulating memories.

how much she enjoyed playing it. From this image, another member of the group shared that she too had enjoyed playing the piano and had forgotten about how significant the joy and pleasure was. By the end of the session, the group had asked the two women if they could play for them, which they did at subsequent meetings. This is one small example of how powerful photographs can be to the memory process.

Listed below are some common uses of images and photographs for creative arts programming:

Distribute pictures from magazines, old calendars, and books for your group to cut up. At the end of every year, card shops place on sale all leftover calendars. This is a great time to stock up because many calendars are photographs of a particular theme. Adaptability is a key in any success-ful group program. Remember, prepare for having participants who are operating at a variety of levels and capabilities within one group. For this type of project, it may be necessary to do some preparatory work; for example, cutting out some photos so that participants who no longer have fine motor skills to operate scissors can easily choose a photo and glue it onto the collage.

The instructions for this type of program can be as simple as asking the participants to choose images that speak to them or as complex as having the participants draw a time line representing their lives and then instructing them to identify photos that can represent the different time periods of their lives. The group also can be directed to use photographs to make a group project such as a wall mural for an upcoming event. Another creative use of photographs is to photograph the participants, glue each photo to the center of a page, and then have each participant create a collage of objects, places, and significant things around the images.

Collages also can be constructed inside boxes. Wooden boxes and paper boxes can be obtained from cigar and cigarette shops; often they will be happy to give them to you for free. Using old or new magazines, ask the group to gather photographs that speak to what their interests are, what they might have owned, or what they still enjoy. Have participants glue photographs onto all sides of the box. This successful program again allows the participants to reminisce while creating an art project. Following are some other ways to use photographs:

- Three-dimensional collages
- Photographing the environment
- Incorporating photographs into two-dimensional artwork
- Incorporating old original photographs into new images by photo-copying the old photographs
- Adding words and poetry to the photographic images

This experience with photographs stimulates the sensory cortex (feeling) in the reaction to what is being photographed. The occipital lobe (seeing) is stimulated by the visualization of the photographic process that participants are experiencing. The reticular formation (arousal) is stimulated by the thought process and positive stimulation of endorphins in the mind and the body. The temporal lobe (hearing) is stimulated by the group's conversations and the voice of the therapist. While the participants share their individual insights, Broca's area (speech) is being stimulated (see Figure 1.4).

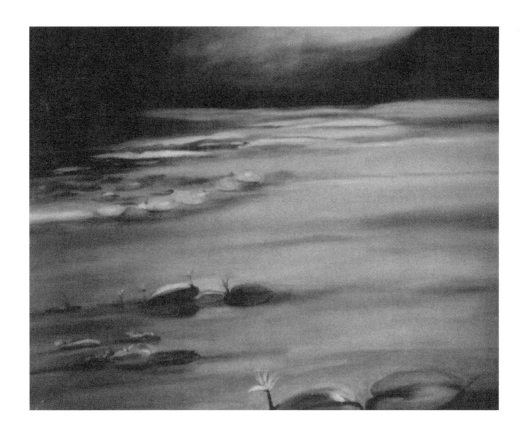

CHAPTER 5

The Continuum of Psychological Domains in Therapeutic Thematic Arts Programming

Why is it that people are so fearful when they begin to think about America's future as an aging society? Part of the reason is surely that many of us are locked into images of decline that are based on outdated impressions of what individual aging entails. Because our social institutions have responded to aging as a problem, we tend to see only losses and overlook opportunities in the process of aging.
—Moody, 1978

DEFINING THE WELL ELDERLY WHO ARE SERVED TODAY

As one walks down the street, anywhere in America, the average age is 55 years and older. The average age of all nursing facility residents across the United States is 87.5 years (National Institutes of Health, 1995). These figures indicate that the aging individuals who are being served today were born between the early 1900s and the mid-1930s. This group is widely known as the pre–World War II generation. The average education commonly was to the sixth grade because the economic responsibilities to the family lay on the shoulders of these children far earlier than in any other generation. These older Americans worked their entire lives and retired at 65 years of age. These factors play a large role in the attitudes these aging Americans have concerning recreation and leisure. It is necessary for a therapist who serves this group to understand that many of the activities that younger generations commonly experienced in elementary and secondary schooling were not experienced by these individuals. Many older Americans have never worked with clay or other common art materials that are used in modern elementary schools (see Figure 5.1). Many have never had leisure time before acquiring a disability.

This phenomenon is slowly changing, because Americans now generally are educated through high school, and attending college is the norm rather than the exception. The increased level of education among older adults might cause future disability rates to drop instead of rise. Studies have indicated that higher levels of education are associated with higher incomes, better nutrition, and better health care (U.S. Census Bureau, 2005). Although the number of older adults who have long-term disabilities has increased, the percentage of the older adults who reported having no disabilities rose during the 1980s. There is reason to believe that older adults who have a higher degree of education also have a greater command of their health and of their free time (Diamond, 1999). Unlike previous generations, the face of aging is changing in many ways, including in the areas of education, leisure awareness, and the importance of managing free time.

To discuss therapeutic recreation programming for well older adults, it is important first to understand the aging individual in this specific point in time along the spectrum of the life span. Many researchers in the field

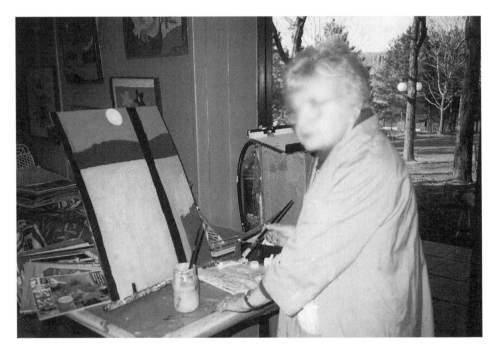

Figure 5.1.   This woman was a social worker, who found painting later in life and exhibited her work in urban art galleries.

of developmental psychology have written about and documented the five domains that directly make up the human existence: the social domain, the emotional domain, the cognitive domain, the physical domain, and now the spiritual domain. These domains are the basic components on which therapeutic intervention can be based when developing individual and group programs. Therapists have always discussed the fundamental principles that each psychological domain encapsulates, yet the concept of using these domains together or separately as significant compositional structures for the development of individual programming needs, goals, and objectives has not been addressed. Thematic programming is constructed and designed by assessing which domain or domains are highlighted for each special group or individual. Later in the chapter, each domain is analyzed for program design.

PSYCHOLOGICAL DOMAINS AS THEY RELATE TO ASSESSMENT OF THE ACCOUNTABILITY MODEL OF SERVICE

The Leisure Ability Model, developed by Peterson and Gunn in 1984 and updated and revised by Stumbo and Peterson in 1998 and 2004 as the Accountability Model of Service, has been well accepted throughout the therapeutic recreation profession. The concept of a continuum of services in the Accountability Model of Service defined and established the differences among functional intervention, leisure education, and leisure participation. According to Peterson and Stumbo (2000), the mission of therapeutic recreation through the Accountability Model of Service is the enhancement of leisure functioning, whereby the therapist identifies in which area the patient is functioning and then creates programming, or services, for that specific area. The authors further stated that if independent leisure functioning is the overall goal or purpose of therapeutic recreation services, then the functional intervention component can and should address functional behavioral areas (emotional, social, cognitive, and physical) that are prerequisites to or a necessary part of leisure involvement and lifestyle.

The four underlying concepts of the Accountability Model of Service are 1) learned helplessness, 2) intrinsic motivation, 3) choice, and 4) flow. These four concepts are paralleled directly by the fundamental theoretical framework of Therapeutic Thematic Arts Programming (TTAP). In the Accountability Model of Service, the emphasis is on the established needs of the client, with each of the services addressing a different need; the services may overlap and change. Expanding on the Accountability Model of Service, the Continuum of Psychological Domains takes the general foundations and gives further structure and definition to each area of functioning, addressing how the four concepts work within each area of any special population.

THE CONTINUUM OF PSYCHOLOGICAL DOMAINS

The Accountability Model of Service did not address how the activity can best meet the social, emotional, cognitive, physical, or spiritual needs of the individual at each stage of wellness. The TTAP approach not only focuses on the overall enhancement of the leisure function but also addresses the clients' specific needs in the five domains (emotional, social, cognitive, physical, and spiritual) by programming directly to those needs. These five domains can be analyzed in each area along the spectrum of aging: well aging, aging in rehabilitation, aging in skilled nursing, and aging with cognitive disabilities. Individuals in various areas of health care have different needs in each domain. Furthermore, each domain can be highlighted and TTAP themes can focus on specific psychological needs. This concept has never been addressed in the provision of therapeutic recreation for older adults. Through the use of TTAP, the therapist can assess and develop the Continuum of Psychological Domains that best meets the participants' needs at different times throughout the continuum and, most important, develop programming that is designed specifically for the emotional, social, physical, cognitive, or spiritual benefit of a client at the particular time and place.

Table 5.1 defines the spectrum of needs at each stage in the aging process. It is important to note that highlighting one domain does not necessarily mean that it is the only psychological focus; the continuum is meant for the therapist to assess the individual further so that he or she can serve the individual to the best of his or her abilities. As one moves from independence to dependence, so, too, does the importance of each domain shift from social to emotional to cognitive to physical to spiritual.

The concept of the Continuum of Psychological Domains is derived from the constructs of the Biopsychosocial Model (Engel, 1977). The biopsychosocial perspective involves an appreciation of a disease or physical condition that not only manifests in terms of pathophysiology but also simultaneously may affect many levels of functioning, from cellular to organ to person to family to society. This biopsychosocial model was the first to provide a broader understanding of the disease process as encompassing multiple levels of functioning, including the therapist–client or the doctor–patient relationship. Engel's model emphasized that change in one area of an individual's life will affect other areas.

The Continuum of Psychological Domains aims to define better the specific psychological, emotional, physical, or cognitive elements within therapeutic recreation programming that would broaden Peterson and Gunn's philosophy. As Engel (1977) stated, disease or a biological change such as aging has social effects that directly or indirectly affect emotional elements, cognitive effects, and psychological concerns. The Continuum of Psychological Domains aims to identify programming needs in each domain so that the therapist can assess the specific needs of the individual

Table 5.1. The Continuum of Psychological Domains

Value	Well elderly	Assisted living	Skilled nursing	Cognitive impairment	Hospice care
5 (high)	Social	Emotional	Cognitive	Physical	Spiritual
4	Emotional	Cognitive	Physical	Spiritual	Cognitive
3	Cognitive	Physical	Social	Cognitive	Emotional
2	Physical	Social	Emotional	Emotional	Social
1 (low)	Spiritual	Spiritual	Spiritual	Social	Physical

The Continuum of Psychological Domains ranked from most important (5) to least important (1) at different life stages in the therapeutic process.

and then design programming specifically for each domain. In the process of normal aging, social interaction directly affects emotional outcomes. Through emotional gratification, we are moved toward cognitive and physical stimulation. This is the basic principle for understanding and incorporating thematic programming into therapeutic domains. Each individual is unique and different; the Continuum of Psychological Domains is designed to be a "jumping off," or starting, point from which the therapist can better assess and design therapeutic interventions.

Robbins (1998) discussed the biopsychosocial developmental process as adaptation maturation, personality structure, relationships formed, and symbolic processing. The domains emotional, social, physical, and cognitive are integrated within and can be correlated directly to the Continuum of Psychological Domains. Aging affects and is affected by emotionality, which comes from personality structure; socialization correlates with relationships formed; and symbolic processing speaks to the significance of the process of creativity. Cognitive and symbolic processing, which directly involve perceptual processes, can be found in artistic creativity as well as language. It now is recognized that enhancing the subjective experience through the arts increases adaptability and an overall sense of well-being.

In the Peterson and Gunn wellness continuum, which fits over the Continuum of Psychological Domains, the bottom left corner represents the ill individual (functional intervention, once called treatment); moving toward the upper right corner (independent leisure participation) represents the well individual. In this concept of programming to the psychological domains, it can be understood that the well aging individual seeks out activity for social and emotional fulfillment (see Figure 5.2).

The Continuum of Psychological Domains for the Well Elderly: Meeting Social and Emotional Needs

Successful therapeutic programming brings together within a therapeutic milieu individuals who have similar needs and interests. This group, the

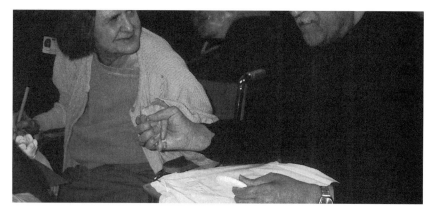

Figure 5.2. Two people find increased socialization through the TTAP method.

well or independent elderly, has experienced many losses, many of them recent, including family members, spouses, occupations, and their own health. The replacement of the once-known social life with a new experience through creative arts, whether it is in an adult day program environment or a community service environment, is fundamental to the overall well-being of the aging individual. TTAP programming for well elders must ensure that the individual will receive social and emotional satisfaction through activities that parallel the importance of the social system and/or family system that the biopsychosocial model describes.

Group events that are developed from individual interests are key to successful participation by well elders. Often at this stage, many changes have occurred and the aging individual finds him- or herself alone and often isolated because past activities no longer are viable and a reinvention of self is required. This reinvention naturally is resisted because of the recurring losses of family and friends that the individual has experienced. The emotional aspects of programming can be facilitated in expressive arts programming.

Allowing the individual, through group activity, opportunities to express his or her inner thoughts, ideas, or conflicts can lead to a greater understanding of the self. This personal positive emotional experience can lead to the reinventing of oneself at the last stage of life. This sense of control has a direct effect on combating learned helplessness and increasing intrinsic motivation through personal choice, which allows the highest levels of flow to exist.

A dominant theoretical approach for viewing the significance of social involvement in human behavior is the ecological systems model (Germain, 1979). This model emphasizes the adaptive fit of humans to the elements of the environment, often referred to as the person in environment. Here, *person* refers to the client system. The client system can be an individual, a family, a group, or a social organization. The environment includes both macro- and micro-level systems as well as resources that are required for sustenance. Social work typically refers to macro and micro as a way of distinguishing levels, big or small (Garvin & Tropman, 1992). Macro-level systems are composed of society, community, and organizations. Micro-level systems in social work are individuals, family, and groups. Long and Holle (1997) further discuss that although each system is intrinsically complete, each relates to the other or may constitute a subsystem of other, larger social sets.

A systems theory approach allows recognition of human behavior as a result of a multiplicity of factors, both internal and external. These factors operate continuously in transition. Individuals not only operate individually but also operate and interact within a larger system of family and community. The individual influences his or her environment, and the environment influences the individual. Therapists must remember to view the individual and his or her behaviors within the context of the environment and the systems that are at work within this environment.

TTAP was developed within the systems approach; each individual is a part of the group, which symbolically represents the family, as discussed by Haynes and Holmes (1994) and Bowlby (1980). This programming also creates an environment that can represent safety and security by creating a place for transformation in which the arts increase adaptability and an overall sense of well-being.

Emotional Needs of the Well Elderly Individual   Csikszentmihalyi's (1990) theory of flow states that when one feels in control of his or her actions, he or she has a true balance of positive emotional experiences through the attainment of competence, enjoyment, and even exhilaration. Even a small gain in control is beneficial, making life more enjoyable and more meaningful (Csikszentmihalyi, 1990). Flow, as conceived by Csikszentmihalyi (1990, 1996), considers all of the creative arts activities the prime "conductors" that meet all of the conditions of this flow, or optimal human experience.

Csikszentmihalyi defined flow as joy, creativity, and the process of total involvement. Flow is achieved by attaining a balance between the extremes of boredom and anxiety by matching appropriate challenges to skills or ability levels. If skills of the individual are not challenged sufficiently, then flow cannot occur and boredom usually results. Challenges are increased to achieve the flow state. Challenging the abilities of individuals through creative arts experiences, if not excessive, represents a more complex emotional experience and results in adjustment and growth (Csikszentmihalyi, 1990). TTAP meets all of the criteria found in what enables the flow process to take place and flourish.

The formula that Csikszentmihalyi described from years of research in the phenomenology of positive experience has the following nine characteristics:

1. Clear goals

2. Feedback regarding process

3. Exercise of skill

4. Intense concentration

5. Diminished awareness of mundane concerns

6. A sense of control

7. A loss of self-consciousness

8. An altered sense of time

9. Enjoyment of the experience for its own sake

These nine characteristics can be accomplished through the TTAP method.

The Continuum of Psychological Domains for Assisted Living: Meeting the Emotional Needs through Social Involvement

Often when an individual moves from independent to dependent living, the emotional aspects are the most difficult. The individual first and foremost is emotionally upset at the element of "the unknown" that is about to occur as he or she moves into a new building with new faces and shares a new room with a total stranger, who most likely is from a different cultural background. The individual has no other choice and has no control over these variables.

Programming to meet these emotional needs can be facilitated through verbal and nonverbal methods; nonverbal communication is important because this type of emotional trauma, moving from all that was known to all that is unknown, is so difficult that the individual often cannot speak about exactly how he or she is feeling. The nonverbal exercises, such as painting, drawing, sculpture, music, and movement, are excellent ways to allow the individual to start to relax into the unknown. The creative arts therapies address the emotional component by providing the individual the opportunities for personal accomplishments and by facilitating independence whenever possible. The emotional component also can be supported by programming to the abilities that the person still has, such as vision, fine motor coordination, and so forth, and accentuating these abilities rather than the disabilities that the individual might be facing, such as overall weakness, fragile physical state, and depression.

The Continuum of Psychological Domains for the Individual in Rehabilitation: Meeting the Physical and Emotional Needs

In the special group of individuals who are in rehabilitation, there is a physical element that must take place for the individual to resume normal daily activities. The individual's physical disability often is sudden and unexpected, such as a car accident, a fall, trauma to the brain, or broken bones. Because of this sudden event, the individual is thrown into a position of dependence on others. The individual who is in physical rehabilitation is best served by a positive and encouraging therapist. The most important requirement for the individual in rehabilitation is to have a strong mind set. The saying "mind over matter" can be a simple way of viewing this special group of individuals. The better one feels emotionally, the quicker the physical recovery; programming to meet the emotional needs of the individual is therefore paramount. The ability to learn a new skill or master an old craft can directly affect the body, mind, and spirit of the individual.

TTAP programming for individuals who are in rehabilitation first should explore and assess the interests that the individual had during his or her life. Interests may come from childhood or adolescence, which might not have been explored in adulthood. These interests now can be central to TTAP. Adaptation is another important element when working with individuals who are in rehabilitation. These individuals often cannot physically function as they had previously. Thus the therapist must adapt activities so that the patient can feel self-challenged, but not to the point of frustration.

The Continuum of Psychological Domains for Individuals in a Skilled Nursing Facility: Meeting the Cognitive and Physical Needs

Individuals who are in a skilled nursing facility (SNF) can have vast and varying needs. Cognitive emphasis is highlighted because research has shown that the more the brain is used in activities, the more alert the mind remains. At another cognitive level, individuals who are completely dependent and have given up their homes and possessions often are depressed. Statistics indicate that more than 65% of nursing facility residents have some form of depression (Vacco, 1998). Accompanying the cognitive needs are the physical needs. Individuals who are in a SNF need modified exercise programming, which requires creative thinking by the therapist. Using the TTAP method, the therapist will want to focus especially on object relations, through which the individual has multiple opportunities for integration of lifetime experiences.

The Continuum of Psychological Domains for the Individual with Dementia: Meeting the Cognitive and Spiritual Needs

Successful thematic programming for individuals with dementia emphasizes and draws from the cognitive abilities that the individual still has left. It is extremely important to focus on what the individual can still do so that frustration does not occur. Dementia takes away so very much of the individual's ability to function that each individual must be assessed for what best can facilitate goals that meet that individual's needs.

Rowe and Kahn (1987) discussed how the quality of life as humans age increases with continued physical and cognitive stimulation. Other research studies (Verghese et al., 2003) have revealed that active older individuals are the least likely to be at risk for cognitive loss such as dementia or Alzheimer's disease (Wilson et al., 2002), depression, cognitive loss, and other physiological problems. The older individual can display working strengths through organized activity and autonomous ego functions, thus being less likely to experience depression and or cognitive loss. Work can be experienced as a pleasurable accomplishment that increases self-esteem and reinforces a distinct certainty about oneself. Despite the lack of research regarding quality of life and aging, Rowe and Kahn (1998) discussed the belief in extrinsic psychological properties that have a positive influence on the overall well-being of older adults. Sterritt and Pokorny (1994) researched the effects that creativity has on elderly individuals diagnosed with dementia who are living in a skilled nursing facility. Findings include decreased heart rate, decrease in medications, and an overall sense of well-being, which directly affects overall quality of life.

Researchers are starting to correlate external stimulation with how cognitive functioning is affected (Rowe & Kahn, 1998). More has been learned about the brain since the early 1990s than in the preceding 85 years (Yankner, 2000). Through technological breakthroughs in modern medicine, researchers are developing a new understanding of the brain's functioning and its ability to regrow cells in the hippocampus and the amygdala. Outward brain stimulation of the right and left brain functions, through reading, writing, and logic (left brain), and through creative art experiences of painting, sculpture, and music (right brain), causes the cells in these regions to rejuvenate and reproduce. These breakthroughs could dramatically affect the understanding of the importance of therapeutic activities throughout the life span as they relate and directly affect *brain wellness* (Diamond, 2000). Significant findings suggest that lack of social interaction through conversation and shared thoughts has a direct cognitive effect on the hippocampus, causing individuals to show signs of further decline in language abilities and short-term memory. TTAP follows the concept of "use it or lose it," stimulating all aspects of brain functioning while also addressing social needs.

THE TTAP METHOD FOR THE WELL ELDERLY INDIVIDUAL

As a model of TTAP at its highest and most complex level, the use of this method with well elders is described here. The following chapter discusses appropriate adaptations and shifts in emphasis for other groups of elders who have compromised abilities.

Understanding where the individual is in the life span is relevant in programming and the integration of powerful life issues that can be rediscovered in the group process. Refer to Erikson's eight stages that were discussed in detail in Chapter 2. The most significant area that is discussed in programming for the well elderly individual is the incorporation of the five domains: social, emotional, cognitive, physical, and spiritual.

When the well elderly individual comes into a group experience, the main area of focus is on the two domains of social and emotional needs. As pointed out by Peterson and Gunn (1984) and updated by Stumbo and Peterson (1998, 2004) and Peterson and Stumbo (2000) in the model of therapeutic services, there can be a movement from independent recreation participation back and forth across the continuum through functional and independent leisure pursuits. The well elderly individual has taken a huge psychological step in walking through the door of the community center, the arts facility, or the adult day program center to restructure once again his or her social systems. This moment can be emotionally charged and therefore possibly can render the individual emotionally and socially vulnerable.

The Social and Emotional Needs that Should Be Emphasized in and Incorporated into the TTAP Method

The ability to be present to others in a group directly reduces boredom while increasing self-worth, which has been written about and researched in the work of Brasile et al. (1997). Emphasizing the individual's responses, the individual's ability to share, and the individual's life, memories, and significant issues are crucial to emotional and social well-being. The individual yearns for social interaction, so the therapist should continually provide the opportunity for social interaction.

The well elderly individual operates in the area of social abilities. The social opportunities that are made available to the individual through TTAP will allow the individual to self-promote emotional well-being, cognitive pursuits, and physical needs.

Following is a list of the nine stages of TTAP with suggested topics for the well elderly individual that emphasize meeting social needs:

Step 1: From individual thought to shared ideas on the page

- Emphasize individual experiences. Ask participants what interests them. Pay attention to the seasons. Is a holiday coming up? Are there any special events in the news? These types of questions provoke the individual to give personal perspectives.

- Vacations or holidays: Ask about vacations that each group member has taken. There will be a lot of positive information shared.

- Family, religion, culture, and traditions: Think about incorporating family tree projects into theme programming; ask about and list brothers, sisters, aunts, and uncles. Simple conversations regarding how color is perceived in various cultures is interesting and informative.

- Life lessons: Everyone can relate to this topic, and the responses will be varied.

- Fashion, movies, and life problems and solutions

Step 2: From ideas on the page to music off the page

- Emphasize music of a specific time period. Most participants will have been born in the 1930s and 1940s, so be prepared for music from the 1950s to be very popular!

- Build on personal music preferences. Often music and specific songs can elicit memories of special people, times, and places. An entire theme can be built around music in general or one particular artist.

- Make musical instruments. This can be a fun project and can foster individual gratification and a sense of accomplishment. One easy way to make musical instruments is to collect cans from home or the kitchen. Have participants paint the cans and then fill them with beans. Different-size beans will elicit different sounds. Cover the opening with a cloth or tape.

Step 3: From the music in the mind to the image

- Emphasize whatever image emerges from the music and build on the image. An example of this is if the participants are playing animal music and then decide to paint jungle scenes.

- Use the active and responsive social abilities that these individuals still have. Continually ask questions!

- If multiple images emerge, then use them in collages, diagrams, or landscapes.

Step 4: From the image into sculpture

- Emphasize familiar images in everyday life. Use flowers, center-pieces, fruit bowls, and other common objects that emerge from the drawing.

- Make sculptures from common objects (see Figure 5.3); it is easy and allows for a certain level of comfort because the object is famil-

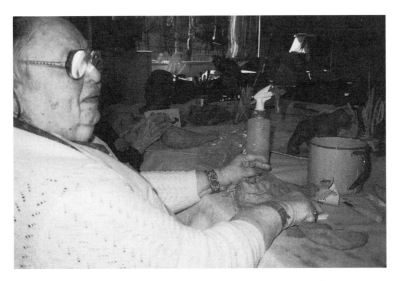

Figure 5.3. A woman who never worked with clay before finds her creative voice.

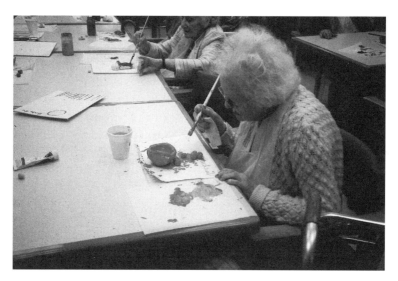

Figure 5.4. This woman is painting a piece of sculpture she created.

iar. For example, if an individual draws flowers, then he or she might want to sculpt the vase and then paint the sculpture that was created (see Figure 5.4).

Step 5: From sculpture into music (kinesthetic)

- Emphasize connecting the thematic approach to what can be used in the movement and dance program. If the participants sculpted flowers, then try to have a discussion of who would be tallest, which flower would move differently, and so forth. If the sculptures incorporated balloons, then bring the balloons into a movement program.

Step 6: From movement into words/poetry and stories (linguistic)

- Emphasize connecting additional words, feelings, and phrases into poetry. If the movement group used fabrics, then ask participants to write down as many colors as they can remember. Then incorporate these colors into the words of a poem.

- Investigate and put down on paper how the individual felt during programming. If the group has been using sounds and reminiscing with musical pieces, then have the participants put down on paper words that describes these feelings that have come up for them.

Step 7: From words into food for thought (linguistic)

- Emphasize connecting the language and words and then using the foods that would fit the theme (see Figure 5.5). If the program is around Valentine's Day, then have a group conversation about which foods can be used to prepare a Valentine's Day celebration.

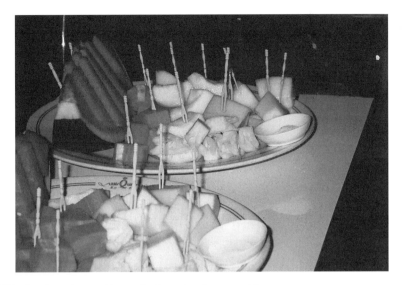

Figure 5.5. Food can be used to emphasize color, shape, and form.

Step 8: From thought into theme event (interpersonal)

- Emphasize connecting all of the links of themes that were derived during the week's program.

- Use the paintings to decorate the walls, the sculptures for center-pieces, and the food to make a meal for the group.

Step 9: From event into photography (intrapersonal)

- Emphasize using photography (see Figure 5.6) to capture each individual for future picture collages and also the event for the group experience.

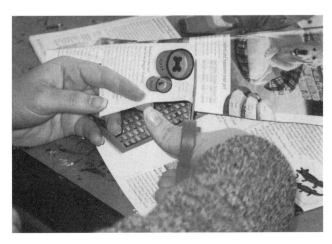

Figure 5.6. Fine motor coordination is used in cutting the photos.

- Use Polaroid and digital photos. Each allows photos to be distributed immediately after they are taken. This immediate gratification can be very rewarding, especially if you are having a family event with relatives.

CONCLUSION

This chapter identified various elderly populations we serve today and highlighted realistic issues that face therapists in health care when providing therapeutic interventions through the creative arts. As discussed, contemporary growth psychology has long accepted the concepts that the five domains—social, emotional, physical, spiritual, and cognition—make up human existence. What affects one area ultimately affects all five domains. The Continuum of Psychological Domains looks to enhance our understanding of these areas and how they interrelate at various stages in the life cycle through sickness and in health.

As therapists we have the responsibility to assess, plan, develop, implement, and evaluate the programming we provide. Hopefully this concept of psychological domains gives a structure and serves as a model for how each specific domain adds to our understanding of how a client's strengths in one psychological domain (e.g., social) can help to overcome the weaknesses in another area (e.g., physical) when confronted with a life change such as, for example, having an accident and being placed in rehabilitation.

Additionally, this chapter identified how the Continuum of Psychological Domains parallels the concept of the Accountability Model of Service in that there are continual leisure and therapeutic experiences through our lives, and this movement through sickness and health can also be reflected in each of the five psychological domains. If we can assess more thoroughly the strengths and weaknesses of our clients, we can define their goals more clearly. Our mission is to create focused, person-centered behavioral interventions to better meet the individual needs of each client. Through the examples provided in this chapter, each domain can be highlighted and a theme can be created to focus on the psychological needs of each individual.

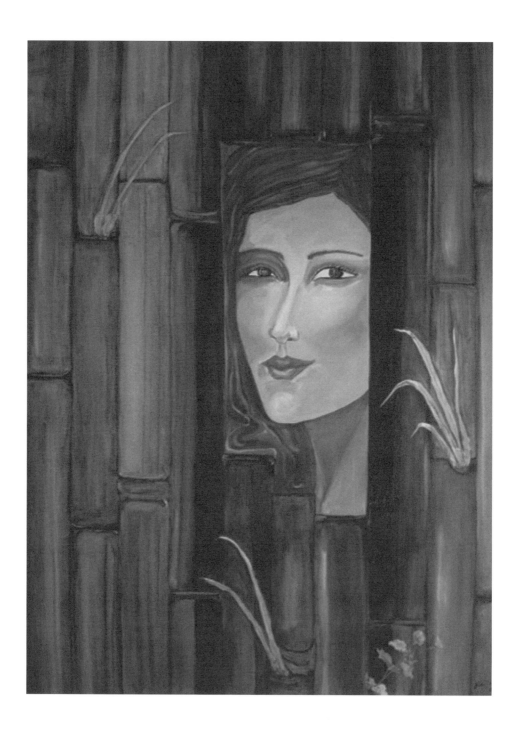

Using Thematic Therapeutic Arts Programming with Older Adults Who Need Assistance

Going into an assisted living facility is like entering outer space. You know it exists on some level, yet you really never wanted to live there.
—Anonymous patient, 1987

Older people who are no longer entirely independent turn to a variety of service settings for the assistance they need in their daily lives. If they are recovering function after an accident, they may stay for a time in a rehabilitation center. If they need assistance on an ongoing basis with activities of daily living, they may move permanently into an assisted living or nursing facility. People with dementia have a unique set of needs due to their cognitive losses and can be found in all levels of long-term care depending on the level of dementia they are experiencing. Therapeutic Thematic Arts Programming (TTAP) can be used effectively with each of these groups of older adults, but the priority of the five psychological domains will vary across service settings. This chapter will look at important variations within the nine steps of the TTAP model that will help a therapist customize the program for each setting as well as for working with people with Alzheimer's disease and other dementias.

A sample TTAP program protocol is provided in Appendix B. It outlines in detail the specific procedures, risks, and outcomes for four of the nine steps in a program designed by the author for individuals diagnosed with early Alzheimer's disease or mild cognitive impairment.

THE TTAP METHOD IN ASSISTED LIVING

Assisted living facilities are the most abundant and fastest growing type of structure being built across the United States (Vacco, 1998) because increasing numbers of older adults are entering this type of facility. To the individuals who are entering assisted living facilities, the quality of the programming is extremely important because they are experiencing tremendous changes. Often these individuals have suffered losses such as death of a loved one and physical losses as a result of aging and becoming more dependent on those around them; on entering an assisted living facility, they also must give up most of their possessions. Close your eyes and think of all of your possessions in every room of your home. Visualize all of these objects: clothing; kitchen utensils; living room and family room furniture; and personal items such as books, musical instruments, and so forth. Then imagine someone telling you that you can keep only what can fit into three 36″ × 36″ boxes; you must decide what goes into these boxes and what you must leave behind.

These individuals are already emotionally traumatized before you as a therapist meet them. Their ability to cope with all of these changes depends on what kind of support systems can be built within the facility. Every person who resides in an assisted living facility has been independent and now must make the adjustment to what could be perceived as being dependent. Sometimes they have to room with someone they might not know, and they now have to eat when told and shower on the nursing schedule.

With these upheavals in mind, the following goals are important to keep in mind when working with older adults in assisted living:

- Enhance residents' quality of life.

- Provide activities that have always been part of the individuals' recreation.

- Provide new and stimulating activities that individuals can learn (see Figure 6.1).

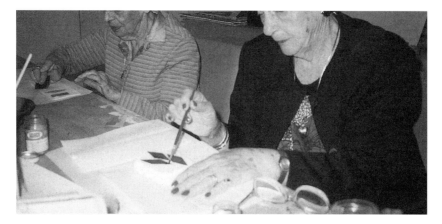

Figure 6.1.   This well older individual is making enamel jewelry for herself; this is an activity that she learned at 80 years old.

- Make residents feel as though this is a good place in which to grow old.

- Foster self-esteem through therapeutic experiences.

- Provide opportunities that allow for self-worth.

- *Motivate, motivate, motivate!*

TTAP can assist these individuals as they learn to cope with all of the changes they are experiencing. Often, the changes experienced by a person who has just moved into an assisted living facility become overwhelming and the individual starts to self-isolate. This can lead to physical decline. For these reasons, the therapist must focus first on the emotional needs and meet the individual where he or she is. If the person is resistant to come to group programming, then the therapist should bring the program into the resident's room in a one-to-one format until a trusting relationship is built. In the Continuum of Psychological Domains in Chapter 5 (see Table 5.1), notice that the first significant value for elders in assisted living is emotional, moving into cognitive. If the individual is supported emotionally, then the social aspects will follow. Keeping in mind this continuum of the five domains allows for a more full understanding of the focus on which TTAP in assisted living should be.

Assisted Living/Rehabilitation
Emotional > Cognitive > Physical > Social > Spiritual

Examples for the nine steps of TTAP in assisted living facilities:

Step 1: From individual thought to shared ideas on the page

Emphasis is on past leisure experiences: vacations, holidays, family, religion, culture, traditions, life lessons, fashion, movies, life problems and solutions, and places where participants never have been or places to which they would like to go back.

Step 2: From ideas on the page to music off the page

Emphasis is on music of the specific time period or music of personal preferences that were derived from and support the theme of step 1. Music can be used as background stimulation and to jump into step 3.

Step 3: From the music in the mind to the image

Emphasis is on building on the image that emerges from the music. Keeping within a theme, residents can paint or draw an object or figure, for example, that represents a country they have visited (see Figure 6.2).

Step 4: From the image into sculpture

Try using themes such as colors or favorite fruit, or bring in a selection of objects for participants to sculpt.

Step 5: From sculpture into music (kinesthetic)

Emphasis is on connecting the thematic approach to what can be used as objects in the movement and dance program: scarves, colorful pieces of fabric, musical instruments, and so forth. Be sure to keep programming at a mature level and to adapt programming to any physical restrictions that the clients might have (if an individual in the group has had professional experience, then let him or her take the lead and teach others; this enhances self-esteem while encouraging others to do the same).

Step 6: From movement into words/poetry and stories (linguistic)

Emphasis is on connecting additional words, feelings, and phrases into poetry. Develop a group poetry session. Participants call out words or phrases that link to the theme. The therapist connects the isolated words into a piece of poetry.

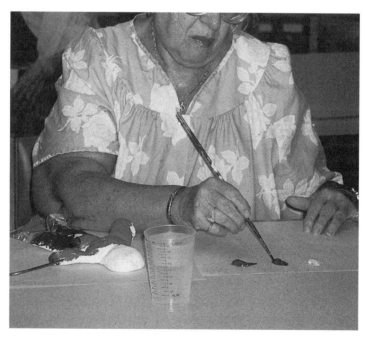

Figure 6.2.   This photograph shows a resident ''in the flow'' process of painting.

Step 7: From words into food for thought (linguistic)

Emphasis is on connecting the language and words and then using the foods that would fit the theme. Cooking groups are extremely successful. Most women have cooked and prepared food their entire lives and enjoy sharing recipes, and many men enjoy cutting and sorting food.

Step 8: From thought into theme event (interpersonal)

Emphasis is on connecting all of the themes that were derived throughout the program and using the paintings to decorate the walls, the sculptures for centerpieces, and the food to make a meal for the group.

Step 9: From event into photography (intrapersonal)

Emphasis is on using photography to capture each individual for future picture collages and also the event for the group experience. These photographs can be used to promote the program; put them in frames and hang them in public areas.

THE TTAP METHOD IN REHABILITATION

As the length of hospital stays has been reduced, short-term rehabilitation settings have become one of the largest health care segments in the U.S. health care system. Short-term goals must be the main focus when programming for this group because the average stay can range from 2 days to sometimes 2 months. Motivation, validation, and reminiscence all are fundamental in short-term rehabilitation.

For an individual who is in a rehabilitation facility, the important elements to be considered are coping with loss, decline in the physical domain, and lack of independence. Therapeutic activities are designed to increase group participation, which automatically enhances social interactions. TTAP should aim to increase a sense of belonging. This can be accomplished just by having each member of the group share an experience, which is extremely important because they suddenly have been taken out of their personal surroundings and brought into a sterile health care environment to accomplish a significant physical task or master a physical disability. Their circumstances decrease self-esteem, self-worth, and a sense of identity and challenges their coping skills.

Following are important goals to keep in mind when working in short-term rehabilitation programs:

* Enhance coping abilities.

* Encourage group participation.

- Enhance sense of well-being.

- Revisit previous interests and accomplishments.

- Provide opportunities for self-awareness.

- Provide steps of a theme that can be completed during stay.

In applying the Continuum of Psychological Domains (see Table 5.1), it is useful to distinguish the two different stages into which the individual in rehabilitation can fall. Rehabilitation can be placed either between the well elderly and assisted living columns or between the assisted living and skilled nursing columns because an individual who enters the rehabilitation facility can move either way on the health continuum, depending on the outcome of the rehabilitation program. Either the individual improves immediately and moves back home within 10 days, or the injury is so severe that the individual starts to decline physically because of age and physical inability to recover.

Well/Rehabilitation
Social > Emotional > Cognitive > Physical > Spiritual

Assisted Living/Rehabilitation
Emotional > Cognitive > Physical > Social > Spiritual

When a therapist assesses an individual who is in rehabilitation, focus should move primarily from emotional to spiritual, because when an individual finds him- or herself suddenly without use of a limb or speech, the emotional element of the person's psyche is crucial for his or her ability to heal mentally and physically. The individual in short-term rehabilitation, however, can fall between the need for social stimulation and emotional needs. The social component will be important, but the individual also has been through a life-altering situation, so that the emotional support is critical. This continuum of domains can change from person to person. For instance, if your client in rehabilitation has multiple sclerosis and makes repeated visits to the rehabilitation facility, then his or her emotional needs will be dramatically different from a teenager who is paralyzed suddenly from a car accident. The Continuum of Psychological Domains is for the therapist to use to evaluate what the primary focus of the therapeutic intervention should be. Keeping in mind this continuum of the five domains allows a more full understanding of the two different domains within which the rehabilitation client can fall and on what the focus of TTAP should be.

Examples for the nine steps of TTAP in rehabilitation settings:

Step 1: From individual thought to shared ideas on the page

Emphasis is on positive individual experiences: Which activities did they do in the past that brought great pleasure? Which movies or books are of interest? What traveling was done with family or friends? The focus moves away from the specific moment in time to when they can recall being happy, satisfied, and fulfilled with life. Past vacations, holidays, family memories, and any other positive experiences should be the primary basis for developing themes.

Step 2: From ideas on the page to music off the page

Emphasis is on music of the specific time period or music of personal preferences that were derived from and support the theme of step 1. Individuals can make musical instruments, or the therapist might explore the future and develop a "wish list," in which activities are created around an object in rehabilitation can be very rewarding; the ability to take home the work is validating. The challenges with short-term rehabilitation will be the time limits of the development of programs; one must look for short, one- or two-session activities.

Step 3: From the music in the mind to the image

Emphasis is on focusing on a place or time when the individual had a problem that he or she overcame. Giving the individual the ability to revisit and reprocess long-term memories is extremely valuable at this stage of life, in this case through drawing, painting, or collage. It also is valuable to share these memories with a group. Often other individuals will share similar issues and solutions. Revisiting a problem that had a clear solution will reinforce each person's belief system. Listening to others tell their stories can be equally rewarding. Remember that the individual in rehabilitation needs to reinvent him- or herself, and having positive reasons to do so can make the process easier. Focusing on when these clients have succeeded or overcome challenges in their pasts will be of great influence.

Step 4: From the image into sculpture

Explore what was drawn or painted, and then turn that into a sculpture. This also can be adapted to something that the individual never had the chance to learn, such as pottery, mosaic tile work, wood work, or wire sculpture.

Step 5: From sculpture into music (kinesthetic)

Emphasis is on connecting the thematic approach to what can be used as objects in the movement and dance program. In addition, use images that can be acted out or that can be embodied in a movement experience. This can be adapted with the help of physical therapy; after the doctor has prescribed therapeutic recreation, the therapist must assess the physical capabilities and disabilities before programming can be planned. Assessment of each client is extremely important to his or her rehabilitation.

Step 6: From movement into words/poetry and stories (linguistic)

Emphasis is on connecting additional words, feelings, and phrases into poetry. How the individual felt during programming can be investigated and put down on paper. Expand on what has been happening to the individual's mind, body, and spirit during rehabilitation. This is a good opportunity to start a journal.

Step 7: From words into food for thought (linguistic)

Emphasis is on connecting the language and words, drawing connections, and then using the foods that would fit the theme. Here again, the individual might want to use words to cope with feelings that are not being expressed or feelings that might need to be written in a journal and not shared.

Step 8: From thought into theme event (interpersonal)

Emphasis is on connecting all of the themes that were derived during the program and now using the paintings to decorate the walls, the sculptures for centerpieces, and the food to prepare a meal for the participants.

Step 9: From event into photography (intrapersonal)

Emphasis is on using photography to capture each individual for future picture collages and also the event for the group experience. This is an excellent event for short stays, which sometimes are only a day or two. An interesting project is to take instant photographs of the clients, cut the image from the background, and then have them draw a background that they wish to invent or visualize. They can finish by pasting themselves into their own vision.

THE TTAP METHOD IN A SKILLED NURSING FACILITY

> *Throughout my childhood and adult life, I took care of my aging parents; coming into this home has given me my first opportunity to live my life.*
> —Anonymous patient, 1989

Moving into a skilled nursing facility (SNF) can be fundamentally one of the most crucial, life-changing events through which an individual can live. The individual gives up all aspects of a private life, including showering in private, eating when hungry, having quiet time alone, and coming and going freely without constraints.

What balances these negative feelings is that most individuals who move into a SNF realize that they cannot take care of themselves at home anymore. The person, therefore, does not resist this dramatic change because it frequently is the only option.

Following are important goals to keep in mind when working in a SNF:

- Engage residents in activities.

- Provide new activities that they might not ever have tried.

- Make residents feel comfortable and at home.

- Foster self-worth and independence through therapeutic experiences.

- Provide opportunities that allow for self-expression.

- *Adapt! Adapt! Adapt!*

Note the pathway for residents of a SNF in the Continuum of Psychological Domains:

Skilled Nursing
Cognitive > Physical > Social > Emotional > Spiritual

Research has shown that the first year in a SNF is the most important for the overall well-being of individuals and their adjustment to a new environment. Cognitive stimulation is crucial for adjustment and continued involvement in the life within the SNF. If an individual turns off mentally, then there often is a dramatic physical result. The physical decline then can lead to spiritual withdrawal and the loss of the will to live.

Cognitive stimulation enhances the individual's fight to survive. It provides reasons to live in a foreign environment. Focusing on cognitive stimulation, the therapist must assess important aspects of the individual's past interests. If a resident was a traveler, then the cognitive exploration of various countries can be a great starting point for thematic programming. If the resident loves books but now cannot read, then the cognitive stimulation can begin with movies or recordings that have been created from a favorite book. These types of cognitive stimulation begin to bridge the gap between a world left behind and the life of today. The therapist can formulate a multitude of themes that can be derived from each of the domains.

One of the most significant elements of the TTAP method is that it allows for the time spent on projects to be increased and one project to be connected to another. Residents in a SNF have time as their advantage. TTAP increases the options for individuals to continue work on their own or to explore varying options within one specific area of the creative arts. For example, if an individual had never painted before, yet during step 3 (from music to the image) found a great talent to draw or paint, then he or she could continue in this one specific creative area of expression.

TTAP provides the therapist with a model that can expand with each new participant and with each new idea that is introduced into the group setting. Creating stimulating programs using continual participation from group members is one of the primary elements in providing the best therapeutic interventions possible.

Examples for the nine steps of TTAP in skilled nursing facilities:

Step 1: From individual thought to shared ideas on the page

Emphasis is on the outside world as well as the world within the SNF. People, places, and times are good themes. Use themes such as seasons; season-appropriate vacations; people in the news; and experiences such as vacations, holidays, family, religion, culture, traditions, life lessons, fashion, movies, and life problems and solutions. Using graphic charts works well with this population.

Step 2: From ideas on the page to music off the page

Emphasis is on music of the specific time period or music of personal preferences that was derived from and supports the theme of step 1. Ask residents to start by naming favorite singers and songs. Soundtracks from movies can foster new thematic ideas that come from group discussion. Rain forest, ocean, or jungle sounds can be excellent sounds from which to create an entire nine-step program.

Step 3: From the music in the mind to the image

Emphasis is on building on the image that emerges from the music. Use the active and responsive social abilities that this group still has. If multiple images emerge, then use them in collages, diagrams, or landscapes.

Step 4: From the image into sculpture

Emphasis is on all types of images, both old and new. The SNF is a place where the individual will grow old. Often, new technology, scientific information, and the arts evolve while the person is living in the SNF; therefore, it is important to bring current events into everyday life in the SNF. This includes providing new and stimulating art materials and mixed media.

Step 5: From sculpture into music (kinesthetic)

Emphasis is on connecting the thematic approach to what can be used as objects in the movement and dance program. Significant in the SNF is the ability to take longer in developing each step of a theme.

The residents have the time to make objects for their musical and movement programs.

Step 6: From movement into words/poetry and stories (linguistic)

Emphasis is on connecting additional words, feelings, and phrases into poetry. How the individual felt during programming can be investigated and put down on paper. This can be facilitated as an individual project or a group project.

Step 7: From words into food for thought (linguistic)

Emphasis is on connecting the language and words and then using foods that would fit the theme. Various cultural foods can be explored.

Step 8: From thought into theme event (interpersonal)

Emphasis is on connecting all of the themes that were derived throughout the program and now using the paintings to decorate the walls, the sculptures for centerpieces, and the food to prepare a meal for the participants. Different types of music can be mixed to create a theme.

Step 9: From event into photography (intrapersonal)

Emphasis is on using photography to capture each individual for future picture collages and the event for the group experience.

THE TTAP METHOD FOR ALZHEIMER'S DISEASE AND OTHER DEMENTIAS

Approximately 4.5 million Americans—one in five of those who are ages 75 to 84 years and nearly half of those who are 85 years and older—have Alzheimer's disease (AD). The National Alzheimer's Association estimates that 15 million people will have AD by 2050 (U.S. Census Bureau, 1997). People with AD represent the largest segment of older adults in institutional settings in the United States. AD is the most common reason for placement of older adults in nursing facilities (Vacco, 1998). These individuals typically live 10 years or longer.

The therapeutic recreation specialist faces the challenge of developing programming to meet the needs of this very special group of clients. One of every three certified recreation therapists will work with older adults, according to the 2005 census taken by the American Therapeutic Recreation Association, and many of these will have memory impairment. Unfortunately, many classes and formal training do not provide real hands-on directives for working with this group of individuals. It has been well established through empirical research that individuals with AD can receive direct benefit from therapeutic recreation programming (Buettner, 1988, 1999; Buettner & Ferrario, 1998; Buettner, Kernan, & Carroll, 1990; Buettner, Lundegren, Lago, Farrell, & Smith, 1996; Buettner & Martin, 1995).

TTAP was first developed for individuals with AD. In the late 1980s through the 1990s there was a complete void as to what type of therapeutic programs could be implemented successfully with this special group. Common questions that psychotherapists and social workers ask regarding residents with AD include the following: Is there programming that could be done? Is the patient able to remember enough to participate in an arts program? What if the client never participated in art? Could they now learn? All of these questions can be answered with one word: *Yes!* The individual with AD can be taught new procedures because this is a function of the brain that is not affected until late in the disease.

> *A therapist was working on a unit with residents who had diagnoses of mild and moderate stages of AD. The thematic program focused on clay sculpture. As the therapist was conducting the group of approximately 15 residents, a couple, who obviously were relatives of someone in the group, entered the back of the day room so as not to disturb the relative. As the therapist continued with the project's instructions and helped the individuals finish their art sculpture, she wondered what the relatives were thinking. Was this project too childlike from a second-party perspective? Would they believe that their relative's abilities were being reduced to that of a 10-year-old? After the residents finished their sculptures, the therapist walked around and asked each member to verbalize what he or she had created. The response was wonderful; each resident came alive verbally, describing what he or she had sculpted and the reasons behind it.*
>
> *At the conclusion of the session, the couple approached the therapist, who prepared herself for a negative comment or two. The husband stated that his mother was one of the members of the group and, to the therapist's surprise, thanked her because, "I have never seen my mother verbalize like she did today, and you made her so happy to participate in this art therapy group" (the therapist, of course, had not made his mother do anything; the older woman had been totally in control). The therapist first was relieved that the couple's response was so positive, but, more important, she realized something that day that reinforces the concepts of thematic programming. The therapist had never known this woman before she became a resident at the facility and did not know that she never spoke or got excited. What the therapist did know was that when the woman was in the group, she was a verbal participant and was obviously reaping the benefits of this type of programming. The therapist believed that the main reason for this success was that she had no preconceived notions about the woman's disabilities* because she was focused only on her *abilities*.

The essence of TTAP programming for individuals with AD lies in the assessment of both the strengths and the weaknesses that emerge within the course of the disease. The therapist then plans the intervention by incorporating the abilities of the individuals into creative arts programming. AD causes a person's communication skills to deteriorate along a somewhat predictable course. This often is one of the largest challenges for the therapist. Deterioration of memory, understanding, speech, language, and social skills takes a toll on a client's ability to communicate effectively. Any therapist who has encountered this group of clients will agree that some days are better than others, and this often is confusing and frustrating for the therapist. TTAP provides some guidelines and helpful tips to prepare the therapist for the frustrating moments that can arise when working with individuals who have this devastating disease.

Caregivers and therapists can better understand the communication behaviors of individuals with AD by realizing not what is lost during the disease process but, more important, what is preserved. Therapists are taught that the success in any therapeutic programming lies in using the abilities that the individual still has and ensuring that frustration, stress, and feelings of incompetence do not arise.

In the early stage of AD, the person starts to experience difficulty with describing short-term events; a productive program, therefore, will develop from choosing a theme from the participants' pasts, such as weddings, and have each person share something about a wedding in which he or she participated or about the person's own wedding. The ability to retrieve long-term memories, such as one's wedding day, is a strength that can be built on in programming. Diamond (1999) confirmed that the ability to recall a positive experience activates the endorphins within the brain, thereby providing positive feelings, regenerating brain cells, and promoting a better quality of life.

Santo Pietro and Ostuni (1997) documented that the ability to structure a sentence properly remains intact until late in the disease. Conversely, some skills, such as word finding, weaken almost from the beginning of the disease. With the right kind of support, the therapist can help the individual find the correct words to describe events.

DEFINITIONS IN AD

It will be helpful for the therapist working with people with dementia to understand some common problems associated with the disease.

Communication Disorder

Communication disorder, which is a condition of communication deterioration, starts from the onset of the disease. It interferes with a person's ability to understand the communication of others. Not understanding speech from others, especially in a group situation, can be very frustrating. It is helpful for the therapist to repeat or clarify the words or phrases of others to ensure that communication breakdown does not occur often.

Communication Breakdown

Communication breakdown occurs when the participant does not understand the words of the speaker at all. Multicultural groups often are found within therapeutic programs, which can be more difficult for participants with AD because of varying dialects and pronunciations. The therapist must be sensitive to tones and word pronunciations to minimize the communication breakdown. Talking slowly and engaging the client through eye contact is important for successful communication. This is a good reason to use the visual word boards (see discussion of this tool in Chapter 4), referring to them often when discussing a topic or a theme.

Learned Helplessness

Learned helplessness, described by Seligman (1975), arises when an individual discovers through repeated experiences that his or her actions have little effect on the outcome of the situation, especially in the "restricted" environment of a nursing facility. Through TTAP, the individual directly affects the group through participation and the act of doing and creating artwork. The involvement of "doing" keeps the client continually feeling positive and valued, thus combating helplessness.

Window of Lucidity

A window of lucidity is a moment when an individual with AD suddenly remembers things or talks more clearly about ideas that seem to have been long forgotten. These can occur very unpredictably, but it is not unusual for them to occur when an individual is engaged in artistic or expressive activities.

Lilly was in the middle stages of AD. She was unaware of where she was, the time of day, and the year. The therapist invited her to join the art group, which was decorating masks. The therapist was not sure that Lilly would be capable, so an aide assisted her. She vigorously decorated her mask with paints and feathers until completed. The therapist then asked the participants to name their masks and discuss any feelings that they had. When it was Lilly's turn, she named her mask after her brother, Ben, and gave a full description of the time when, as a child, Ben found a pack of matches and set fire to his crib. He was fine but needed to wear a bandage on his face for a while. Lilly then showed the group where she had placed a piece of tissue paper that represented the bandage that her brother had had to wear. When Lilly's daughter came to pick her up that day, the therapist asked about the story that Lilly had told the group. The daughter had not been aware of this event and said that she would ask her uncle. The next day, Lilly's daughter confirmed that in fact Ben had set fire to his crib.

COMMUNICATION AS THE FIRST STEP IN TTAP

As discussed by Santo Pietro and Ostuni (1997), communication breakdown is common in meeting the treatment and socialization needs of individuals with AD. Individuals who have AD are struggling with the following seven issues, and being sensitive to these concerns enables better participation, less frustration, and more successful communication:

1. Loss of independence

2. Loss of social roles

3. Loss of physical attractiveness and grooming skills

4. Loss of energy

5. Loss of family and friends

6. Loss of familiar environments

7. Loss of first-language partners

Similarly important to note is that certain abilities are preserved until later stages of AD and should be incorporated into TTAP. They include

1. The use of procedural memories

2. The ability to retrieve early life memories

3. The ability to recite, read aloud, and sing with good pronunciation

4. The ability to engage in social rituals

5. The desire for interpersonal communication

6. The desire for interpersonal respect

The Use of Procedural Memories

The individual with AD begins to lose memory for words, information, and events, but procedural memory, which is the knowledge of how to perform tasks, remains relatively intact until the late stages of dementia. Scientists have defined procedural memory as the most elemental of human memory systems that exist in the executive region of the brain and are capable of operating independently. Anderson (1990) explained that procedural memory is like a computer program; other types of memories are like separate forms of memory data stored within the computer. Individuals who are in the middle stages of AD do not know where they are going, but they remember how to walk. They do not wash their own clothes anymore, but give them fabric, soap, and water and they will wash. Similarly, they might not know what they are saying, but they still can speak.

Specific examples of procedural memories include folding clothes, pouring, setting the table, washing hands, and passing plates. TTAP incorporates procedural memories into thematic programming. The themes *food* and *facts* illustrate how to emphasize procedural memories.

Food is one of the most essential elements of life, starting from birth and ending at death. Food as a theme is an excellent focal point for using procedural memories for individuals with AD.

1. Discuss which types of food are eaten for various meals. Plan a meal with the participants. This can include designing a menu, choosing the foods, and, most significant, preparing food. The use of plastic utensils is important. Cutting foods such as bananas, melons, and breads is easy, and the participant derives much pleasure from the successful event.

2. Counting is another interesting and creative way to use food. String beans; peanuts; jelly beans; and apples, pears, and any other fruit with seeds can be distributed among the participants, and then participants can be instructed to count objects or the seeds. Make this a challenge game, and give prizes for the winner. Next, have participants cut up the food for a salad or to cook.

3. Food for Thought is a simple activity that asks the group to think about various foods and then add personal stories that are related to the foods. Cultural foods such as Chinese dim sum, Jewish pastries, Cuban rice and beans, and Italian ices or fresh mozzarella and tomatoes can be used for this type of procedural activity.

Use of the theme of *facts* can be stimulating in many different ways.

1. Using the visualization board, ask participants to list facts about a common item, such as clothes. Have participants list various components of clothing, such as buttons, zippers, clasps, and so forth, then bring in samples of these components and have participants operate the items.

2. The theme of facts also can be specific to performing tasks. Have participants visualize how they dance or exercise. Then have them act out the movements of these familiar acts. Revisiting old memories is significant to the overall well-being of the participants.

The Ability to Retrieve Early Life Memories

The earliest memories seem to be held deep within the brain, and they resist deterioration until late into the disease process. In addition, it has been proved that the memory of positive experiences can affect the immune system, psychological well-being, and overall quality of life. Butler (1963) asserted that life review is a valuable tool with which older adults can leave a legacy, thus increasing feelings of self-worth and self-esteem. The Life Review Program, developed by Tabourne (1991, 1995), follows Erikson, Erikson, and Kivnick's (1986) revision of Erikson's original theory and integrates Butler's theory into a cognitive approach to cognitive skill development and memory work with older adults with mild to moderate dementia. The themes *memories* and *life lessons* illustrate how to emphasize early life memories.

Overall, the important goals to keep in mind when working with people with Alzheimer's disease are to

- Enhance residents' quality of life.

- Provide activities that the residents can still do.

- Allow residents a feeling of control over their environment.

- Foster self-worth through therapeutic experiences.

- Provide opportunities that allow for self-expression.

Medical research into the deterioration caused by dementia has found that the need to keep mentally active is the key to slowing the progression of cognitive deterioration. With this in mind, it makes sense to start programming in the physical domain where the individual still feels capable of following simple directions and deriving great pleasure from socializing within a group.

Cognitive Impairment
Physical > Spiritual > Cognitive > Emotional > Social

Spiritually, the residents continue to reach out to the philosophies and religious beliefs that they have known their entire lives. Moving into cognitive thematic programming again brings in recreational interests that the residents have had their entire lives. Thus, leading the resident through TTAP ensures a rich, socially stimulating process.

Step 1: From individual thought to shared ideas on the page

Emphasis is on individual experiences from the past: vacations, holidays, family, religion, culture, traditions, life lessons, fashion, movies, and life problems and solutions. Again, the visual word board is an excellent visual reminder for this group of individuals, who may experience difficulties processing language in spoken form.

Step 2: From ideas on the page to music off the page

Emphasis is on music of the specific time period or music of personal preferences that were derived from and support the theme of step 1. This population flourishes with musical stimulation. Play a piece of music from a favorite movie or Broadway show.

Step 3: From the music in the mind to the image

Emphasis is on building on the image that emerges from the music. Use the active and responsive social abilities that these individuals still have. If multiple images emerge, then use them in collages, diagrams, and landscapes.

Step 4: From the image into sculpture

Emphasis is placed on any form of abstract art made with clay, wire, or paper. There are no "mistakes"; everything created is of value.

Step 5: From sculpture into music (kinesthetic)

Emphasis is on connecting the thematic approach to what can be used as objects in the movement and dance program. In addition, use images that one can act out or can be embodied in a movement experience. For example, participants can act out "being" a tree in a wind storm.

Step 6: From movement into words/poetry and stories (linguistic)

Emphasis is on connecting additional words, feelings, and phrases into poetry. Any feelings that come to mind can be put down on paper. For example in a movement program related to the wind, participants can act out how trees move in the wind. Then the therapist can write down on the board (discussed in Chapter 4) any words that the group can think of in relation to the wind (e.g., cold, bitter, wild, scary) and then link these words by using rhyming or storytelling.

Step 7: From words into food for thought (linguistic)

Emphasis is on connecting the language and words and then using the foods that would fit the theme. Revisit some examples for using food for counting, remembering social events, or cultural stimulation.

Step 8: From thought into theme event (interpersonal)

Emphasis is on connecting all of the themes that were derived throughout the program and using, for example, the paintings to decorate the walls, the sculptures for centerpieces, and the food to make a meal for the participants.

Step 9: From event into photography (intrapersonal)

Emphasis is on using photography to capture each individual for future picture collages and the event for the group experience.

CONCLUSION

More and more in today's society, a person's age is truly *just a number*. Individuals are living longer through better nutrition, health, and skin care and are continually redefining what old age is and what it looks like. We now see famous older celebrities, such as Lauren Hutton, look into the camera and state, "This is what 60 looks like." Betty Friedan (1999) was the first individual to redefine what *old* is, describing three concepts: *young old* (65–75 years old), *old old* (75–85 years old), and *oldest old* (85–100+ years old). It is the author's belief that a new era has begun in which people will live an entire life in old age. Women are expected to live well into their 100s through advancements in modern medical and scientific technology. In the early-1990s, an 80-year-old having hip replacement surgery would have been unusual; now it is commonplace.

As life expectancy is continually redefined, so will new developmental periods emerge that move beyond Erikson's (1982) "Integrity versus Despair." The increase of time will provide moments to reminisce, share in group conversations, revisit past pleasures, and partake of new experiences that will enhance this additional psychological stage of old age. For now, individuals going into a SNF could live an additional decade or two. The therapist in health care will become increasingly important in providing, through person-centered thematic programming, opportunities for this complicated stage of integration versus despair to develop and unfold. By providing creative therapeutic interventions, health care therapists will enhance lifetime experiences through these leisure experiences. Providing multiple opportunities to revisit the past, integrate the past with the present, and look into the future, the role of the creative arts therapist is central to the facilitation of psychological wellness and emotional fulfillment during these last stages of life.

In the final analysis, aren't people more truly themselves during their leisure and free time than at any other time of their daily lives?

TTAP provides an important opportunity for older adults in a variety of settings to enjoy this full expression of self and the many benefits that can result. This book has demonstrated how TTAP can be used effectively in populations including well elderly and people with dementia, and with patients or residents in rehabilitation, assisted living, and skilled nursing care facilities.

- There are nine steps for all populations.

- The Continuum of Psychological Domains relates to each population.

- TTAP can help meet the needs of health care regulations in the 21st century.

- Endless creativity in programming can develop from the TTAP format.

TTAP provides person-centered programming that is relevant to the individual's past and then moves that experience into the present during programming.

Contact Dr. Levine Madori regarding how you have used this new method or other questions at Linda@Levinemadoriphd.com.

References

American Psychiatric Association. (1994). *Diagnostic and statistical manual of mental disorders, 4th edition* (DSM-IV). Washington, DC: Author.

Anderson, J. (1990). *The adaptive character of thought.* Hillsdale, NJ: Lawrence Erlbaum Associates.

Anderson, S., Ball, S., Murphy, R.T., et al. (1975). *Encyclopedia of educational evaluation.* San Fransisco: Jossey-Bass.

Auerbach, J., & Benezra, A. (1998). Therapeutic recreation and the rehabilitation of the stroke patient. In W. Sife (Ed.), *After stroke: Enhancing quality of life* (pp. 123–128). New York: Hawthorne Press.

Austin, D. (2001). *Therapeutic recreation: Processes and techniques.* New York: Sagamore Publishing.

Avedon, E.M. (1974). *Therapeutic recreation service: An applied behavioral science approach.* Englewood Cliffs, NJ: Prentice Hall.

Baltes, P.B., & Willis, S.L. (1982). Plasticity and enhancement of intellectual functioning in old age: Penn State's Adult Development and Enrichment Project (ADEPT). In F.I.M. Craik & S. Trehub (Eds.), *Aging and cognitive processes* (pp. 353–389). New York: Plenum Press.

Baltes, P.M., & Baltes, M.M. (1990). Psychological perspectives on successful aging: The model of selective optimization with compensation. In P.M. Baltes & M.M. Baltes (Eds.), *Successful aging: Perspectives from behavioral sciences* (pp. 1–34). New York: Cambridge University Press.

Baltes, P.M., Reese, H.W., & Lipsitt, L. (1980). Life span developmental psychology. *Annual Review of Psychology, 31,* 65–110.

Bandura A. (1997). *Self-efficacy: The exercise of control.* New York: W.H. Freeman.

Bandura A. (2001). Social Cognitive Theory: An agentive prespective. *Annual Review of Psychology, 52,* 1–26.

Barrett, C.E. (1986). In search of brain–behavior relationships in dementia and the Lauria-Nebraska neuropsychology battery. In E.D. Taira (Ed.), *Physical and occupational therapy in geriatrics: Current trends in geriatric rehabilitation* (pp. 113–139). New York: Haworth Press.

Bloom B.S. (Ed.). (1956). *Taxonomy of educational objectives, Handbook 1: The cognitive domain.* New York: David McKay Co.

Bowlby, J. (1980). *Attachment and loss, Vol. 3: Loss and sadness, and depression.* New York: Basic Books.

Brasile, F.M., Hendrick, B.N., Manny, B., Haussy, P., Legernes, K., & Prathipati, S. (1997). Efficacy of an interactive computer game in physiological and psychological outcomes related to arm ergometer exercise participation of hospitalized elderly patients. *Annual in Therapeutic Recreation, 7,* 52–63.

Bright, R. (1988). *Music therapy and the dementias: Improving the quality of life.* St. Louis: MMB Publications.

Broach, E., Groff, D., Dattilo, J., Yaffe, R., & Gast, D. (1997–1998). Effects of aqua therapy on adults with multiple sclerosis. *Annual in Therapeutic Recreation, 7,* 1–20.

Brotons, M., & Marti, P. (2003, Summer). Music therapy with Alzheimer's patients and their family caregivers: A pilot project. *Journal of Music Therapy, 40*(2), 138–150.

Buettner, L.L. (1988). Utilizing developmental theory and adaptive equipment with regressed geriatric patients in therapeutic recreation. *Therapeutic Recreation Journal, 22*(3), 72–79.

Buettner, L.L. (1999, July). Simple pleasures: A multilevel, sensorimotor intervention for nursing home residents with dementia. *American Journal of Alzheimer's Disease,* 137–142.

Buettner, L.L., & Ferrario, J. (1998). Therapeutic recreation-nursing team: A therapeutic intervention for nursing home residents with dementia. *Annual in Therapeutic Recreation, 7,* 15–26.

Buettner, L.L., Kernan, B., & Carroll, G. (1990). Therapeutic recreation for frail elders: A new approach. *Global Therapeutic Recreation I* (pp. 82–88). Columbia, MO: University of Missouri Press.

Buettner, L., Lundegren, H., Lago, D., Farrell, P., & Smith, R. (1996). Therapeutic recreation as an intervention for persons with dementia and agitation: An efficacy study. *American Journal of Alzheimer's Disease, 12*(4), 1–8.

Buettner, L., & Martin, S.L. (1995). *Therapeutic recreation in the nursing home.* State College, PA: Venture.

Butler, R. (1963). The life review: An interpretation of reminiscence in the aged. *Psychiatry, 26,* 65–76.

Caldwell, L.L., Dattilo, J., & Kleiber, D.A. (1994–1995). Perceptions of therapeutic recreation among people with spinal cord injury. *Annual in Therapeutic Recreation, 5,* 134–125.

Coatman, C. (1996). *Thanks for the memories: Alzheimer's disease—The insidious assassin.* Irvine, CA: University of California Irvine Research and Treatment Center.

Coghill, R. (2000). *Exploring the nervous system: Brain imaging.* Retrieved April 2, 2003, from http://Faculty.Washington.edu/chudler/image.html

Cohen-Mansfield, J., Werner, P., & Rosenthal, A. (1992). Observational data on time use and behavior problems in nursing homes. *Journal of Applied Gerontology, 11*(1), 111–121.

Csikszentmihalyi, M. (1990). *Flow: The psychology of optimal experience.* New York: Harper & Row.

Csikszentmihalyi, M. (1996). *Creativity: Flow and the psychology of discovery and invention.* New York: Harper Perennial.

Dattilo, J. (2000). *Facilitation techniques in therapeutic recreation.* State College, PA: Venture Publishing.

Dattilo, J., & Hoge, G. (1994–1995). Perceptions of leisure by adults with mental retardation. *Annual in Therapeutic Recreation, 5,* 27–37.

Deci, E.L. (1975). *Intrinsic motivation.* New York: Plenum.

Deci, E.L., & Ryan, R.M. (1985). *Intrensic motivation and self deternmination in human behavior.* New York: Plenum Press.

DeMong, S.A. (1997). Provision of recreational activities in hospices in the United States. *Hospice Journal, 12*(4), 57–67.

Diamond, M. (2000). *Older brains and new connections.* San Luis Obispo, CA: Davidson Publications.

Donovan, J. (1996). Exploratory-level dramatherapy within a psychotherapy setting. In S. Mitchell (Ed.). *Dramatherapy: Clinical studies* (pp. 91–107). London: Jessica Kingsley Publishers.

Dunn, N., & Wilhite, B. (1997). The effects of a leisure education program on leisure participation and psychosocial well-being of two older women who are home-centered. *Therapeutic Recreation Journal, 31*(1), 53–73.

Edgington, C.R., Jordan, D.J., DeGraaf, D.G., & Edgington, S.R. (1998). *Leisure and life satisfaction: Foundational perspectives* (2nd ed.). Boston: McGraw-Hill.

Engel, G.L. (1977). *The need for a new medical model: A challenge for biomedicine. Science, 196*(4286), 129–136.

Erikson, E.H. (1963). *Childhood and society* (2nd ed.). New York: W.W. Norton.

Erikson, E.H. (1982). *The life cycle completed: A review.* New York: W.W. Norton.

Erikson, E.H., Erikson, J.M., & Kivnick, H.Q. (1986). *Vital involvement in old age.* New York: W.W. Norton.

Folstein, M., Folstein, S., & McHugh, P. (1975). Mini-mental state: A practical model of grading the cognitive status of patients for the clinician. *Journal of Psychiatric Residence, 12,* 189–198.

Gardner, H. (1997). *Extraordinary minds: Portraits of exceptional individuals and an examination of our extraordinariness.* New York: Basic Books.

Garvin, C.D., & Tropman, J.E. (1992). *Social work in contemporary society.* Englewood Cliffs, NJ: Prentice Hall.

Germain, C. (Ed.). (1979). Social work practice: People and environment, an ecological perspective. New York: Columbia University Press.

Golomb, J., Kluger, A., de Leon, M.J. (1996). Hippocampal formation size predicts declining memory performance in normal aging. *Neurology, 47,* 810–813.

Gulick, E.E. (1997). Correlates to quality of life among persons with multiple sclerosis. *Nursing Research, 46(6),* 305–311.

Haynes, K.S., & Holmes, K.A. (1994). *Invitation to social work.* New York: Longman.

Heywood, L.A. (1978). Perceived recreative experience and relief of tension. *Journal of Leisure Research, 10,* 86–94.

Huitt, W., & Hummel, J. (2003). Piaget's theory of cognitive development. *Educational Psychology Interactive.* Valdosta, GA: Valdosta State University.

Iso-Ahola, S.E. (1980). *The social psychology of leisure and recreation.* Dubuque, IA: Wm. C. Brown.

Kelly, J.R. (1996). *Leisure* (3rd ed.). Boston: Allyn & Bacon.

Kennedy, R. (2006). *The emotions and health.* The Doctors' Medical Library. Santa Rosa, CA (http://www.medical-library.net/sites/framer.html?/sites/_emotions.html)

Kraus, R. (1978). *Recreation and leisure in modern society.* Santa Monica, CA: Goodyear Publishing.

Langer, E.J., & Rodin, J. (1976). The effects of choice and enhanced personal responsibility for the aged: A field experiment in an institutional setting. *Journal of Personality and Social Psychology, 34,* 191–198.

Lemonick, M.D., & Park, A. (2001, May). The nun study: How one scientist and 678 sisters are helping unlock the secrets of Alzheimer's. *Time Magazine, May 14,* 55–64.

Levine Madori, L. (2004). Therapeutic recreation participation, cognitive functioning, and psychosocial well-being of skilled nursing facility residents diagnosed with mild or moderate Alzheimer's disease. *Dissertation Abstracts International (UMI No. 3124953)*.

Long, D.D., & Holle, M.C. (1997). *Macro systems in the social environment*. Belmont, CA: Wadsworth Publishing.

Mannell, R.C., & Kleiber, D.A. (1997). A social psychology of leisure. State College, PA: Venture Publishing.

McClellan, T. (2001). Study and analysis of cognitive, motivational and group treatment of alcoholics through brain imaging. *Journal of American Medical Association, 9*, 50–56.

McCluskey, K.A., & Reese, H.W. (Eds.). (1984). *Life span developmental psychology: Historical and generational effects*. Orlando, FL: Academic Press.

Mobily, K. (1985). A philosophical analysis of therapeutic recreation: What does it mean to say "we can be therapeutic"? *Therapeutic Recreation Journal, 19*, 16–17.

Moody, R.A. (1978). *Reflections on* Life After Life. New York: Bantam.

Nation, J.M., Benshoff, J.J., & Malkin, M.M. (1996). Therapeutic recreation programs for adolescents in substance abuse treatment facilities. *Journal of Rehabilitation, 62*, 10–16.

National Institutes of Health. (1995). *Alzheimer's disease: Unraveling the mystery* (NIH Publication No. 95-3782). Silver Spring, MD: ADEAR Printing Office.

National Therapeutic Recreation Society. (1982). *Philosophical position statement*. Alexandria, VA: Author.

Nordoff, P., & Robbins, C. (1977). *Creative music therapy*. New York: John Day.

Peterson, C.A., & Gunn, S.L. (1984). *Therapeutic recreation program design: Principles and procedures*. Englewood Cliffs, NJ: Prentice Hall.

Peterson, C.A., & Stumbo, N.J. (2000). *Therapeutic recreation program design* (3rd ed.). Boston: Allyn & Bacon.

Phillips, B.E. (1956, May/June). Can we agree? *Journal of Health, Physical Education, and Recreation, 27*(5), 52.

Piaget, J. (1952). *The origins of intelligence in children*. New York: International University Press.

Pinderhughes, E.B. (1988). Significance of culture and power in the human behavior curriculum. In C. Jacobs & D.D. Bowles (Eds.), *Ethnicity and race: Critical concepts in social work* (pp. 152–166). Silver Spring, MD: National Association of Social Workers.

Reisberg, B., Ferris, S.H., de Leon, M.J., & Crook, T. (1982). The Global Deterioration Scale for assessment of primary degenerative dementia. *American Journal of Psychiatry, 139*, 1136–1139.

Reisberg, B., & Kluger, A. (1998). Assessing the progression of dementia: Diagnostic considerations. In C. Salzman (Ed.), *Clinical geriatric psychopharmacology* (pp. 432–462). Baltimore: Williams & Wilkins.

Robbins, A. (1998). *Therapeutic presence*. London: Jessica Kingsley Publishers.

Rowe, J.W., & Kahn, R.L. (1998). *Successful aging*. New York: Pantheon Books.

Rubin, D.C. (1995) *Memory in oral tradition*. New York: Oxford University Press.

Santo Pietro, M.J., & Ostuni, E. (1997). *Successful communication with Alzheimer's disease patients*. Boston: Butterworth-Heinemann.

Scarmeas, N., Levy, G., Tang, M.-X., Manly, J., & Stern, Y. (2001). Influence of leisure activity on the incidence of Alzheimer's disease. *Neurology, 57,* 2236–2242.

Schultz, D. (1977). *Growth psychology: Models of the healthy personality.* New York: D. Van Nostrand.

Seligman, M.E.P. (1975). *Helplessness: On depression, development, and death.* San Francisco: W.H. Freeman.

Selman, J. (1988). Music therapy with Parkinson's disease, *British Journal of Music Therapy, 2,* (1), 5–10.

Shivers, J., & Fait, H. (1975). *Therapeutic and adapted recreational services.* Philadelphia: Lea & Febiger.

Siegel, D. (1999). *The developing mind: How relationships and the brain interact to shape who we are.* New York: Guilford Press.

Skalko, T.K. (1990). Discretionary time use and the chronologically mentally ill. *Annual in Therapeutic Recreation, 1,* 9–14.

Snowdon, D. (2001). *Aging with grace: What the Nun Study teaches us about leading longer, healthier, and more meaningful lives.* New York: Bantam.

Stern, Y., Albert, S., Tang, M-X., & Tsai, W-Y. (1999). Rate of memory decline in AD is related to education and occupation: Cognitive reserve? *Neurology, 53,* 1942–1947.

Stern, Y., Gurland, B., Tatemichi, T., Tang, M. X., Wilder, D., & Mayeux, R. (1994). Influence of education and occupation on the incidence of Alzheimer's disease. *Journal of the American Medical Association, 271,* 1004–1010.

Stern, Y., Moeller, J.R., & Anderson, K.E. (2000). Different brain networks mediate task performance in normal aging and Alzheimer's disease: Defining compensation. *Neurology, 55,* 1291–1297.

Sterritt, P.F., & Pokorny, M.E. (1994). Art activities for patients with Alzheimer's and related disorders. *Geriatric Nursing: American Journal of Care for the Aging, 15*(3), 155–159.

Stumbo, N.J., & Peterson, C.A. (2004). *Therapeutic recreation program design: Principles and procedures* (4th ed.). San Francisco: Pearson Benjamin Cummings.

Tabourne, C.E.S. (1991). The effects of a life review recreation therapy program on confused nursing home residents. Topics in *Geriatric Rehabilitation 7*(2), 13–21.

Tabourne, C.E.S. (1995). The benefits of a life review program for a patient newly admitted to a nursing home: A case study. *Therapeutic Recreation Journal, 29*(3), 228–236.

Torres-Rivera, E., Wilbur, M.P., Roberts-Wilbur, J., & Phan, L. (1999). Group work with Latino clients: A psycho educational model. *Journal for Specialists in Group Work, 24,* 383–404.

U.S. Department of Labor, Bureau of Labor Statistics. (2006). *Occupational outlook handbook (OOH), 2006–2007* Edition. Retrieved March 1, 2006, from http://www.bls.gov/oco/

U.S. Census Bureau. (1997). *Government records and statistics: Summary type file 1A.* Washington, DC: U.S. Government Printing Office.

U.S. Census Bureau. (2005). *65+ in the United States: 2005.* Washington, DC: U.S. Government Printing Office.

Vacco, D. (1998, July). *New York State Attorney General's Commission on the Quality of Care at the End of Life. Final report.* Washington, DC: New York State Commission on the Quality of Care at the End of Life.

Verghese, J., Lipton, R., Katz, M., Hall, C., Derby, C., Kuslansky, G., et al. (2003). Leisure activities and the risk of dementia in the elderly. *The New England Journal of Medicine, 348*(25), 2508–2516.

Voelkl, J.E., Galecki, A.T., & Fries, B.E. (1996). Nursing home residents with severe cognitive impairments: Predictors of participation in activity groups. *Therapeutic Recreation Journal, 30(1)*, 27–40.

Voelkl, J.E., & Mathieu, M. (1995). Intra-individual variation in the subjective experiences of older adults in a nursing home. *Therapeutic Recreation Journal, 29(2)*, 114–123.

Warr, P. (1993). Work and mental health: A general model. In F. la Ferla & L. Levi (Eds.), *A healthier work environment.* Copenhagen: World Health Organization.

Weiss, C.R., & Kronberg, J. (1986). Upgrading therapeutic recreation service to the severely disoriented elderly. *Therapeutic Recreation Journal, 20*(1), 34.

Williams, J.R., & Hollan, J.D. (1981). The process of retrieval from very-long-term memory. *Cognitive Sciences, 5*, 87–119.

Wilson, R.S., Mendes de Leon, C.F., Barnes, L.L., Schneider, J.A., Bienias, J.L., Evans, D.A., et al. (2002). Participation in cognitively stimulating activities and risk of incident Alzheimer disease. *The Journal of the American Medical Association, 287*(6), 742–748.

Winnicott, D.W. (1965). *The maturation processes and the facilitating environment.* London: Hogarth Press.

Yankner, B. (2000, March). A century of cognitive decline. *Nature, 404,* 125.

Zatz, M.M., & Goldstein, A.L. (1985). Thymosins, lyphokines and the immunology of aging. *Gerontology, 31,* 263–277.

Zgola, J.M. (1987). *Doing things: A guide to programming activities for persons with Alzheimer's disease and related disorders.* Baltimore: The John Hopkins University Press.

Suggested Readings

Ackerman, S. (1992). *Discovering the brain.* Washington, DC: National Academy Press.

Anthony, E.J., & Benedek, T. (Eds.). (1975). *Depression and the human experience.* Boston: Little, Brown.

Bahrick, H.P., Bahrick, P.O., & Wittlinger, R.P. (1976). Fifty years of memory for names and faces: A cross section approach. *Journal of Experimental Psychology: General, 104,* 54–75.

Bandura, A., Ross, D., & Ross, S. (1961). Transmission of aggression through imitation of aggressive models. *Journal of Abnormal and Social Psychology, 63,* 575–582.

Barnet, A.B., & Barnet, R.J. (1998). The house of meaning. In *The youngest minds: Parenting and genetic inheritance in the development of intellect and emotion* (pp. 28–54). New York: Touchstone.

Bear, M.F., Conners, B.W., & Paradiso, M.A. (1996). *Neuroscience: Exploring the brain.* New York: Lippincott Williams & Wilkins.

Bloom, B.S. (1986). Automaticity: The hands and feet of genius. *Educational Leadership, 43*(5), 70–77.

Bruner, J. (1986). Value presuppositions of developmental theory. In L. Cirillo & S. Wapner (Eds.), *Value presuppositions in theories of human development.* Hillsdale, NJ: Lawrence Erlbaum Associates.

Bush, C.A. (1995). *Healing imagery and music: Pathways to the inner self.* Portland, OR: Rudra Press.

Butler, R.N., & Lewis, M.I. (1982). *Aging and mental health* (3rd ed.). St. Louis: Mosby.

Carter, R. (1998). *Mapping the mind.* Los Angeles: University of California Press.

Cowen, W.M. (1979). The development of the brain. *Scientific American, 241*(3), 106–117.

Davis, J. (1997). *Mapping the mind: The secrets of the human brain and how it works.* Secaucus, NJ: Carol Publishing Group.

Diamond, M., Hopson, J., & Diamond, M.C. (1998). *Magic trees of the mind: How to nurture your child's intelligences, creativity, and healthy emotions from birth through adolescence.* New York: E.P. Dutton.

Feil, N. (1982). *Validation: The Feil Method.* Cleveland, OH: E. Feil Prod.

Fox, J.H. (1977). Effects of retirement and former work life on women's adaptation to old age, *Journal of Gerontology, 32,* 196–202.

Gardner, H. (1980). *Artful scribbles: The significance of children's drawings.* New York: Basic Books.

Gardner, H. (1981). *Quest for mind.* New York: Basic Books.

Gardner, H. (1982a). *Art, mind, and brain.* New York: Basic Books.

Gardner, H. (1982b). *Development of human psychology.* New York: Basic Books.

Gazzaniga, M. (1997). *Conversations in the neurosciences.* Cambridge, MA: MIT Press.

Gazzaniga, M. (1998). *The mind's past.* Berkeley: University of California Press.

Geiger, C.W., & Miko, P. S. (1995). Meaning of recreation/leisure activities to elderly nursing home residents: A qualitative study. *Therapeutic Recreation Journal, 2,* 131–138.

Gersie, A., & King, N. (1990). *Storymaking in education and therapy.* London: Jessica Kingsley Publishers.

Goldstein, E. (1995). *The ego and its function.* New York: The Free Press.

Gwyther, L. (1985). *Care of Alzheimer's patients: A manual for nursing home staff.* Chicago: American Health Care Association and Alzheimer's Association.

Halpern, G.C. (1994). Healing art: Cross-cultural connections. In *Body and soul: Contemporary art and healing.* Exhibition catalogue, DeCordova Museum, Lincoln, MA.

Havinghurst, R.J. (1963). Successful aging. In R. Williams, C. Tibbits, & W. Donahue (Eds.), *Processes of aging* (Vol. 1, pp. 299–320). New York: Atherton Press.

Havinghurst, R.J. (1968). A social psychological perspective on aging. *The Gerontologist, 8,* 67–71.

Havinghurst, R.J., Munnichs, J.M.A., Neugarten, B.L., & Thomae, H. (Eds.). (1969). *Adjustment to retirement: A cross-national study.* New York: Humanities Press.

Havinghurst, R.J., Neugarten, B., & Tobin, S. (1968). Disengagement and patterns of aging. In B.L. Neugarten (Ed.), *Middle age and aging* (pp. 161–172). Chicago: University of Chicago Press.

Heal, M., & Wigram, T. (Eds.). (1993). *Music therapy in health and education.* London: Jessica Kingsley Publishers.

Helmes, E., Caspo, K., & Short, J. (1987). Standardization and validation of the Multidimensional Observation Scale for Elderly Subjects (MOSES). *Journal of Gerontology, 42*(4), 395–405.

Jennings, S. (1994) The theatre of healing: Metaphor and metaphysics in the healing process. In S. Jennings, A. Cattanach, S. Mitchell, A. Chesner, & B. Meldrum (Eds.), *The handbook of dramatherapy* (pp. 93–113). London: Routledge.

Jung, C. (1959). *The meaning of death.* New York: McGraw-Hill.

Kara, D., & Yoels, W.C. (1982). *Experiencing the life cycle: A social psychology of aging.* Springfield, IL: Charles C Thomas.

Kastenbaum, R. (1968). Perspectives on the development and modification of behavior in the aged: A developmental-field perspective. *Gerontologist, 8,* 280–284.

Keller, C., & Fleury, J. (2000). *Health promotions for the elderly.* London: Sage Publications.

Kempermann, G., & Gage, F. (1999). New nerve cells for the adult brain. *Scientific American, 280*(6), 48–53.

Kensington, K. (1970). Psychological development and historical change. *The Journal of Interdisciplinary History, 2,* 329–345.

Kitwood, T. (1997). *Dementia reconsidered.* Buckingham, England: Open University Press.

Levy-Warren, M. (1996). *The adolescent journey: Development, identity formation, and psychotherapy.* Northvale, NJ: Jason Aronson.

Longres, J.F. (2000). *Human behavior in the social environment* (3rd ed.). Itasca, IL: Peacock.

Lynott, R.J., & Lynott, P.P. (1996). Tracing the course of theoretical development of the sociology of aging. *The Gerontologist, 36,* 749–760.

Manis, J., & Meltzer, B. (1972). *Symbolic interaction.* Boston: Allyn & Bacon.

Neisser, U. (1994). Intelligence: Knowns and unknowns. *The American Psychologist, 51,* 77–101.

Neugarten, B.L. (1973). Personality changes in later life: A developmental perspective. In C. Eisdorfer & M.P. Lawton (Eds.), *The psychology of adult development and aging.* Washington: American Psychological Association.

New York State Department of Health and Cabrini Medical Center. (1999/2000). *Education and environment: The effects on Alzheimer's disease.* Research in progress.

Novosad, C., & Thoman, E. (1999). Stability of temperament over the childhood years. *American Journal of Orthopsychiatry, 69*(4). 457–464.

Piaget, J. (1937, 1954). *Piaget cognitive-stage theory. Theories of development.* New York: Freeman and Co.

Piaget, J. (1985). *The equilibrium of cognitive structures.* Chicago: University of Chicago Press.

Pilisuk, M. (2000). A job and a home: Social networks and the integration of the mentally disabled in the community. *American Journal of Orthopsychiatry, 50,* 782–788.

Powell, W. (1998). The ties that bind: Relationships in life transitions. Social casework. *Journal of Contemporary Social Work, 69*(9), 539–540.

Priefer, B.A., & Gambert, S.R. (1984). Reminiscence and life review in the elderly. *Psychiatric Medicine 2,*(1), 91–100.

Runyan, W.M. (1984). *Life histories and psycho biography.* New York: Oxford University Press.

Sachs, P.R. (1995). Marital adjustment to life changes associated with aging. In G.R. Weeks & L. Hof (Eds.), *Integrative solutions: Treating common problems in couples therapy.* Levittown, PA: Brunner/Mazel.

Schaie, K. (1965). Age changes and age differences. *Gerontologist, 7,* 128–132.

Siegel, K., & Freud, B. (1994). *Parental loss and latency age children.* Westport, CT: Auburn House.

Simonette, C. (1978). *Getting well again.* Los Angeles: Jeremy P. Tarcher.

Tabourne, C. (1995). The life review program for an older adult newly admitted to a nursing facility: A case study. *Therapeutic Recreation Journal, 29*(3), 228–240.

Teagle, M.L., McGhee, V.L., & Hawkins, B.A. (1996). Geriatric practice. In D.R. Austin & M.E. Crawford (Eds.), *Therapeutic recreation: An introduction* (2nd ed., pp. 227–244). Boston: Allyn & Bacon.

Toner, J.A., Teresi, J.A., Gurland, B.J., & Tirumalasetti, F. (1999). The feeling-tone questionnaire: Reliability and validity of a direct patient assessment screening instrument for the detection of depression symptoms in cases of dementia. *Journal of Clinical Geropsychology, 14,* 63–77.

Van Andel, G., & Potoven, D. (1995). Case histories focusing on clients with depression: Practical issues. *Therapeutic Recreation Journal, 29*(1), 254–258.

Wald, J. (1983). Alzheimer's disease and the role of art in treatment. *American Journal of Art Therapy, 22,* 57–64.

Warshaw, G., Gwyther, L., Phillips, L., & Koff, T. (1996). *Alzheimer's disease: An overview for primary care.* Tucson: University of Arizona Health Sciences Center.

Weiskopf, D. (1982). *Recreation and leisure: Improving the quality of life* (p. 22). Boston: Allyn & Bacon.

44444444444444444444444444444444444444444444444444444444444444444444444444444444444444444444444444444 stop

Weiss, C.R. (1989). T.R. and reminiscing: The pursuit of elusive memory and the art of remembering. *Therapeutic Recreation Journal, 23*(3), 7–18.

White, L.A. (1994). The concept of culture. In: *Encyclopædia Britannica* (Vol. 16, pp. 874–881). Chicago: Encyclopædia Britannica, Inc.

White, R.W. (1960). Competence and the psychosexual stages of development. *Nebraska Symposium on Motivation, 8,* 97–141.

Williams, J.R. (1995). Using story as a metaphor, legacy and therapy. *Contemporary Family Therapy, An International Journal 17,* (1), 9–16.

Williams, M., & Jones, T. (1990). *Predicting functional outcome in older people. Principles of geriatric medicine.* New York: McGraw-Hill.

Winnicott, D.W. (1980). *Playing and reality.* Harmondsworth, England: Penguin Press.

Wurtman, R.J. (1985). Alzheimer's disease. *Scientific American, 252*(1), 62–74.

Yesavage, J., & Brink, T. (1983). Development and validation of geriatric screening scale: A preliminary report. *Journal of Psychiatric Residency, 17,* 37–49.

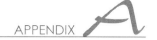

Program Protocols for Therapeutic Thematic Arts Programming

Tapping into Creativity

PROGRAM PROTOCOL 1: WEEK/SESSION 1

Treatment Modality

Meditation and Guided Imagery using *thematic* music and verbal conversation

Rationale

Guided imagery is a way in which to calm the mind and allow thoughts, both past and present, to surface. Using music, the group leader speaks slowly to the residents while they are contemplating the sounds in the music. This program allows residents to freely access their long-term memory by listening to any particular music theme. If the music theme is sounds of the ocean, once participants have listened, a group discussion is stimulated and encouraged by the group leader. Residents share past experiences of places they have traveled. Reminiscing helps the individual review positive and significant experiences had over the course of a lifetime.

This group experience instills a sense of overall positive well-being and increases social stimulation through verbalizing past experiences. Scientists are realizing that the brain responds exactly the same way when revisiting a positive event in thought or in action. Guided imagery is a direct way to use the power of creative imagination in a way that can be immediate and more effective than critical thinking.

Referrals

This program is specifically designed for individuals diagnosed with early Alzheimer's disease or mild cognitive impairment (MCI). Referrals to this program can be

- Self-referral
- Referral by the staff
- Referral by a family member
- Referral by a nurse or companion

Risk Management

This program does not present any organizational risk. However, when reviewing memories, there is a concern that a bad memory might be triggered. Additionally, there might be memories that are too personal to share with the entire group. The recreation therapist must be aware of each participant's responses and be ready to support, comfort, or control any sad or uncomfortable memories that might arise.

Structure Criteria

The initial *thematic music choice* and guided imagery should be no longer than 10 minutes. This will allow residents to become familiar with listening to music and allowing images to come into the "mind's eye" (e.g., sounds of the surf, beach theme; sounds of a tropical forest, animal theme; sound of wind, autumn theme).

The second thematic choice of music should be the same theme, but allow the residents, if comfortable, to listen for a longer period of time. This process of becoming familiar with guided imagery is very common and usually takes only one or two sessions to get used to.

After the residents have listened to the music, start a conversation with open-ended questions. The length of this group can range from 25 minutes to a full hour, including listening to music.

Each module includes

5 minutes of introductions of group leader and participants

5 minutes of explanation of what music will be heard

10 minutes of music playing (residents may close their eyes, if they prefer)

15–30 minutes of discussion, using a blackboard to list ideas and memories that are shared

Process Criteria

The group leader will never leave residents unattended. If any one of the group members gets agitated or upset, another staff member should immediately take him or her out of the group. The group leader will continually encourage quiet listening during the music and conversation after the music is heard.

Each module, the *Therapist* will

Set up the CD/tape player

Instruct residents on how to "listen" to music, with or without eyes closed

Comfort residents who might be in need

Encourage discussion of the music theme

Outcome Criteria

Residents will readily access memories of past experiences. This process works extremely well with residents with MCI, due to their ability to access and then speak about thoughts that surface. The increased socialization throughout the group should be noticeable. This experience allows individuals who normally would not share in conversation to do so through reminiscence and positive sharing experiences in a group.

Each module, the *Resident* will

Be able and be encouraged to express ideas or thoughts about the music

Socialize within the group around the theme presented

Contribute to what is recorded by the group leader

Have multiple opportunities to share feelings and accomplishments with colleagues and reflect on the past

Credentialing

This program should be supervised by Certified Therapeutic Recreation Specialists (CTRS) and conducted by group leaders who have been trained.

Bibliography

Guided Imagery. (2000–2005). Eupsychia Institute. http://www.eupsychia.com/perspectives/imagery.html

National Institute of Aging. (2005, August). *Alzheimer's fact sheet.* U.S. Department of Health and Human Resources. http://www.nia.nih.gov/alzheimers/publications/adfact.html

Alternative Medicine Online. (1998). *Therapies: Meditation therapy.* http://library.thinkquest.org/24206/meditation-therapy.html

Alternative Medicine and Health. (2000). *Meditation Therapy.* Boynton, NJ. http://alternative-medicine-and-health.com/therapy/meditation-therapy.htm

Whole Health MD. (2000). *Meditation.* Sterling, VA. http://www.wholehealthmd.com/ME2/dirmod.asp?sid=17E09E7CFFF640448FFB0B4FC1B7FEF0&nm=Reference+Library&type=AWHN_Therapies&mod=Therapies&mid=&id=7936709D16B94C8F9960E53BCF52C6E7&tier=2

Supplies

Two to three pieces of thematic music

CD (or tape) player

PROGRAM PROTOCOL 2: WEEK/SESSION 2

Treatment Modality

Thematic Painting and Collage Program

Rationale

Working from the ideas that were shared in the first session, the leader will use painting as a thematic approach to the theme of autumn, changes, colors of nature, and so forth. Art helps residents to express their emotions and show creativity. According to *The Ultimate Art Guide*, "The creative arts are a collection of disciplines whose principal purpose is the output of material that is compelled by a personal drive and echoes or reflects a message, mood, and symbolism for the viewer to interpret." The themes portrayed through therapeutic types of music will encourage relaxation and enhance the residents' ability to recall long-term memories which are still very accessible in the first stages of Alzheimer's. Researchers have found that art is a way to restore and even add to one's self-identity as well as to help individuals interpret images for problem solving, conflict, and resolution in the last stages of life.

Referrals

Referrals to this program can be

- Self-referral
- Referral by the staff
- Referral by a family member
- Referral by a nurse or companion

Risk Management

Residents will be using nontoxic paint, although scissors will need to be special-ordered with easy grips and with dull tips to ensure safety. The leader will not leave the group at any time during the program to ensure guidance and safety. Residents might experience frustration, at which time the leader will aid and assist.

Structure Criteria

The initial music session utilized music and guided imagery. This second session will revisit the themes that emerged after the first session by looking at the board or large pad that the leader used to collect group ideas. The leader also will bring music back into the group. Residents will be given painting paper (18 × 24 inches) and asked to paint scenes that come to mind and were reflected in the sharing during the first session. Selection of nontoxic, water-soluble colored paints should be limited to no more than six colors. Participants also will be given pictures of birds to be incorporated into the program.

Each module includes

5 minutes of introductions of the group leader and participants and reflections on the last session

5 minutes of directions on what materials will be used (photographs/paint)

25 minutes of listening to music while painting some recollections of the past

10 minutes of discussion to share what was painted

15 minutes of cleanup

Process Criteria

The group leader will never leave residents unattended. If any one of the group members is getting agitated or upset, he or she should be immediately taken out of the group by another staff member. The group leader will continually encourage painting and the use of photographs while listening to quiet music in the background.

Each module, the *Therapist* will

Set up the CD/tape player

Instruct residents on how to use the paints (demonstration)

Instruct about how to apply photographs to the painted image

Encourage discussion of the final project

Clean up and organize all supplies

Outcome Criteria

Residents will be reminded of the first session, accessing once again the memories of past experiences. Residents will create a painting, with or without the use of photographs, to create an art project to their satisfaction.

Each module, the *Resident* will

Be encouraged to remember thoughts and ideas shared during the first session

Have multiple opportunities to work with paints and/or with photographs

Demonstrate or express feelings of accomplishment

Share thoughts, feelings, and his or her project with others

Reflect on the past

Reflect on positive memories through the art process

Credentialing

This program should be supervised by CTRS and conducted by group leaders who have been trained.

Bibliography

TeBeest, R., Kornstedt, K., Feldmann, C., & Harmasch, L. (2002). *The use of expressive arts in various occupational therapy settings.* http://murphylibrary.uwlax.edu/digital/jur/2002/tebeest-kornstedt-feldmann-harmasch.pdf

Supplies

18 × 24-inch paper

Six choices of tempera paint (nontoxic)

Scissors to cut collage materials

Pictures of birds to be added to paintings

PROGRAM PROTOCOL 3: WEEK/SESSION 3
Treatment Modality

Thematic Sculpture Program: Rain Sticks

Rationale

This program utilizes a peer setting to provide socialization, reinforcement of past art experience, and stimulation of cognitive abilities through enhancing opportunities to interact. The art experience additionally allows the residents to engage in the exploration of objects and materials which, through a thematic approach, encourages self-expression in a nonthreatening shared group experience. The very act of tapping into one's inner resources empowers each resident while promoting feelings of mastery and increased self-esteem. The ability to make something out of raw materials is an enjoyable act at any age. This group experience allows for enhancing memory, orientation, and communication on many levels. The group leader stimulates orientation by continually linking activities. Stimulation of memories is continual as the group leader uses open-ended questions while residents are involved in the sculpture activity. Each resident will create a musical instrument, which will be utilized in a movement program during the next session. The leader should witness enhanced levels of communication among residents.

Referrals

Referrals to this program can be

- Self-referral
- Referral by the staff
- Referral by a family member
- Referral by a nurse or companion

Risk Management

Residents will be using nontoxic paint, scissors, and cardboard tubing. The leader will not leave the group at any time during the program to ensure guidance and safety. Residents might experience frustration, at which time the leader will aid and assist.

Structure Criteria

The initial music session utilized music and guided imagery. This session will revisit the themes that emerged after the first session by looking at the board or large pad that the leader used to collect and write down group ideas. The leader will bring music back into the group and reorient the group to the themes of autumn, rain, and changing weather. Participants will be shown a finished rain stick, which is the instrument they will create.

Each resident will be given a 12-inch hollow cardboard tube and a selection of colorful yarn (which will be limited to 6 colors to avoid frustration with choice).

Each module includes

5 minutes with the group leader reflecting and summarizing the past sessions

5 minutes of directions on how to build a rain stick using the materials shown

25 minutes of winding colorful yarn around the tube to create designs

Leader will assist individuals when needed and will facilitate conversation during the session

5 minutes of sharing each other's creations

10 minutes of cleanup

Process Criteria

The group leader will never leave residents alone or unattended. If any one of the group members is getting agitated or upset, he or she should be immediately taken out of the group by another staff member. The group leader will continually encourage stimulating conversation, movement to the rhythm of the music, and gross motor and fine motor coordination.

Each module, the *Therapist* will

Set up the CD/tape player

Revisit and reflect on the last session

Demonstrate the rain stick already constructed

Demonstrate and hand out materials to individuals

Encourage discussion of the object and its origin

Organize and clean up supplies

Outcome Criteria

Residents will be encouraged to recall what happened in the last session. Residents will again reflect on past experiences and socialize with others. Residents will be encouraged to create, with assistance, a personal rain stick to be used in the following sessions.

Each module, the *Resident* will

Be encouraged to remember thoughts and ideas shared during the first session

Have multiple opportunities to work with yarn, using fine motor coordination, and to socialize with others about the project or self

Demonstrate or express feeling of accomplishment

Share thoughts, feelings, and his or her project with others, and reflect on the past

Reflect on positive memories through the art process

Credentialing

This program should be supervised by CTRS and conducted by group leaders who have been trained.

Bibliography

Col, J. (1998). *Enchanted Learning: Instructions—Rain Stick.* http://www.enchanted learning.com/crafts/music/rainstick/http://ieeexplore.iee.org/xpl/freeabs-all
Barth, K. (2003). *Melodies of the mind: How music works in therapy.* YC24, a production of the New Media Workshop at the Columbia University Graduate School of Journalism. http://nyc24.jrn.columbia.edu/2003/issue3/story2/page2.html

Supplies

Hollow tubes made of cardboard

Six choices of tempera paint (nontoxic)

Six colorful yarns to decorate tube

Heavy brown paper

Foil

Glue

Small dried beans or pasta

Scissors to cut materials

Music in background

PROGRAM PROTOCOL 4: WEEK/SESSION 4

Treatment Modality

Thematic rain sticks used in movement and music session

Rationale

This program utilizes music and movement through the individual instrument the resident made in the previous session. Knowledge of music and its positive effects on people with Alzheimer's disease is continually growing. Clinical studies (Cash, 2006) document the fact that patients who can no longer recognize loved ones can still recall music of their generation. A study in Barcelona, Spain (Brotons & Marti, 2003) found that 14 residents with mild Alzheimer's disease improved in social and emotional areas after receiving music therapy. Music enhances quality of life and simultaneously stimulates thoughts and feelings long forgotten (Health, 2001). This program is designed to increase feelings of self-esteem, socialization, and feelings of self-worth while utilizing a musical instrument that was hand-made during a previous session. Cognitive functioning is stimulated through repetition of directives regarding movement to the music, encouraging participation in a nonthreatening atmosphere while the focus is on the object and not on the individual.

Referrals

Referrals to this program can be

- Self-referral
- Referral by the staff
- Referral by a family member
- Referral by a nurse or companion

Risk Management

Residents will be using rain sticks made in the previous session. The leader will not leave the group at any time during the program to ensure guidance and safety. Residents might experience frustration, at which time the leader will aid and assist.

Structure Criteria

Leader will bring music back into the group and reorient participants to the theme of autumn, rain, weather changes, and so forth. Participants will be asked to bring their rain sticks, which they created in the previous session. The stick is an instrument that creates soothing sounds and will be utilized with music as a tool to create rhythmic movement as well as music. The leader will combine movement with rhythm, thus enforcing the use of the rain stick, the body, and gross motor coordination.

Residents will use body movement and their rain sticks, changing sticks with each other for physical, social, and cognitive stimulation.

Each module includes

5 minutes of introductions and reflection by the group leader and participants on the previous session

5 minutes of directions on the materials to be used, music, movement, and the rain stick

5 minutes of music, encouraging movement to music, alternating with the use of each resident's rain stick. Music with a strong rhythm works best.

10 minutes of discussion regarding sharing the rain sticks and listening to the different sounds each one makes

5 minutes of cleanup

Process Criteria

The group leader will never leave residents unattended. If any one of the group members is getting agitated or upset, he or she should be immediately taken out of the group by another staff member. The group leader will continually encourage stimulating conversation, movement to the rhythm of music, and gross and fine motor coordination.

Each module, the *Therapist* will

Set up the CD/tape player

Instruct residents on how to use the rain stick as an instrument

Demonstrate each movement, slowly and using repetition

Encourage participation

Encourage discussion during the music program by asking open-ended questions

Keep enactments interactive and stay away from solo activity as much as possible

Give residents time to react, because they may be slower to process directions

Outcome Criteria

Residents will be reminded of the initial session, accessing once again the memories of past experiences. Residents will use the musical instrument that they made and be physically stimulated by movement to the music during the program.

Each module, the *Resident* will

Be encouraged to remember thoughts and ideas shared during the first session

Have multiple opportunities to work with yarn, using fine motor coordination, and socialize with others about the project or him- or herself

Demonstrate or express feeling of accomplishment

Share thoughts, feelings, and the project with others, and reflect on the past

Reflect on positive memories through the art process

Credentialing

This program should be supervised by CTRS and conducted by group leaders who have been trained.

Bibliography

Col, J. (1998). *Enchanted Learning: Instructions—Rain Stick.* http://www.enchanted learning.com/crafts/music/rainstick/
http://ieeexplore.iee.org/xpl/freeabs-all

Barth, K. (2003). *Melodies of the mind: How music works in therapy.* YC24, a production of the New Media Workshop at the Columbia University Graduate School of Journalism. http://nyc24.jrn.columbia.edu/2003/issue3/story2/page2.html

Supplies

Previously made rainsticks

CD or tape player

Selection of music for movement

Activity Assessment Form for Therapeutic Thematic Arts Programming

Give a brief description of activity, including individuals served:

Check which learning style this activity encompasses:
(Activity can encompass more than one learning style)

_____ Linguistic learner (the word player)

_____ Logical learner (the questioner)

_____ Spatial learner (the visualizer)

_____ Musical learner (the music lover)

_____ Kinesthetic learner (the mover)

_____ Interpersonal learner (the socializer)

_____ Intrapersonal learner (the individual)

PHYSICAL ASPECTS

1. What is the primary body position required?

   prone _____ kneeling _____ sitting _____

   standing _____ sedentary _____

   other: _____

2. Which parts of the body are required?

   arms _____ neck _____

   hands _____ head _____

   legs _____ upper torso _____

   feet _____ lower torso _____

3. Which types of movement does the activity require?

bending _____ catching _____

stretching _____ throwing _____

standing _____ hitting _____

walking _____ skipping _____

reaching _____ hopping _____

grasping _____ running _____

punching _____

4. Coordination between parts and movements;

1   2   3   4   5

Low   High

5. Eye–hand coordination:

1   2   3   4   5

Low   High

6. Strength:

1   2   3   4   5

Low   High

7. Speed:

1   2   3   4   5

Low   High

8. Endurance:

1   2   3   4   5

Low   High

9. Energy:

1   2   3   4   5

Low   High

10. Flexibility:

1   2   3   4   5

Little   Much

11. Degree of cardiovascular activity involved:

1   2   3   4   5

Little   Much

SOCIAL ASPECTS

1. Interaction pattern regarding person and object (check only one pattern):

Person/object _____

Person/person _____

Object/object _____

Interaction pattern within the activity (check only one):

_____ intraindividual: Action takes place within the mind or action involves the mind and a part of the body.

- requires no contact with another person or external object

_____ extraindividual: Action directed by a person toward an object.

- requires no contact with another person

_____ aggregate: Action directed by a person toward an object while in the company of other people who also are directing action toward objects.

- action is not directed toward each other
- no interaction between participants is required

_____ interindividual: Action of a competitive nature directed by one person toward another

_____ unilateral: Action of a competitive nature among three or more people, one of whom is an antagonist or "it."

- interaction is in simultaneous competitive relationship.

_____ multilateral: Action of a competitive nature among three or more people with no one person as an antagonist.

_____ intragroup: Action of a cooperative nature by two or more people intent on reaching a mutual goal.

- action requires positive verbal or nonverbal interaction

_____ intergroup: Action of a competitive nature between two or more intragroups.

2. Interaction with others

Physical contact: **1**   **2**   **3**   **4**   **5**
    Little   Much

Competition: **1**   **2**   **3**   **4**   **5**
    Little   Much

Emotional response: **1**   **2**   **3**   **4**   **5**
    Little   Much

ADAPTATION TO INDIVIDUALS WITH COGNITIVE IMPAIRMENT

(Check one or more where appropriate)

_____ Mild cognitive impairment

_____ Moderate cognitive impairment

_____ Severe cognitive impairment

COGNITIVE ASPECTS

1. How many rules are there?

1   **2**   **3**   **4**   **5**
Few   Many

2. How complex are the rules?

1   **2**   **3**   **4**   **5**
Simple   Complex

3. How much long-term is necessary?

1   **2**   **3**   **4**   **5**
Little   Much

4. How much immediate recall is necessary?

1   **2**   **3**   **4**   **5**
Little   Much

5. How much strategy does the activity require?

    1   2   3   4   5

    Little   Much

6. How much verbalization of thought process is required?

    1   2   3   4   5

    Little   Much

7. How much concentration is required?

    1   2   3   4   5

    Little   Much

AFFECTIVE ASPECTS

1. Rate the opportunities for the expression of the following emotions during this activity:

	Never			Often	
Joy	**1**	**2**	**3**	**4**	**5**
Guilt	**1**	**2**	**3**	**4**	**5**
Pain	**1**	**2**	**3**	**4**	**5**
Anger	**1**	**2**	**3**	**4**	**5**
Fear	**1**	**2**	**3**	**4**	**5**
Frustration	**1**	**2**	**3**	**4**	**5**

SENSORIAL COMPONENT

1. What are the primary senses required for the activity?

    Rate: 0 = not at all, 1 = rarely, 2 = occasionally, 3 = often

    touch _____

    taste _____

    sight _____

    hearing _____

    smell _____

ADMINISTRATIVE ASPECTS REGARDING THE THERAPIST

1. Leadership: specific activity-skill expertise   _____

   general activity-skill ability   _____

   supervisory   _____

   none needed   _____

2. Equipment: none required   _____

   specific commercial product   _____

   can be made   _____

3. Facilities: none required   _____

   specific natural environment   _____

   specific human-made environment _____

4. Duration: set time   _____

   natural end   _____

   continuous   _____

5. Participants: any number   _____

   fixed number or multiple   _____

Sources for Art Supplies and Music

CREATIVE THINKING WHEN BRAINSTORMING PROJECTS

Look Around the Art Room

Often, when a therapist starts a new position in a facility, the only direction is toward a supply closet. More often than not, the closet has leftover supplies—some still usable, some that a therapist might not ever have used before. If the therapist is lucky, the supplies can suffice until his or her order is processed. A teaching exercise for therapy students is to have them bring to class four or five supplies that have no relation to each other and have them come up with as many projects for as many groups of clients as possible. The goal for students is to become acquainted with creative thinking, or what is commonly known as *thinking outside the box.*

Common Items and What to Do with Them

Old Clay   Clay easily can be made workable again by wetting a towel, twisting most of the water out of it, and wrapping it around the clay. Cover this with a plastic bag for a day or two, and the result will be workable clay and play dough. Play dough can be used on paper to create forms and shapes; this works well with individuals with communication problems.

Popsicle Sticks   The use of sticks can be very inexpensive yet very creative. Participants can make frames for artwork or photographs, bird houses, and flower sculptures.

Pipe Cleaners   Pipe cleaners now come in great colors and assorted sizes. They can be used to create bracelets and necklaces, as hair on clay animals, or in a group project in which everyone attaches his or her pipe cleaner to another person's, creating a huge string. This is a safe and simple material to use.

Colored Paper   Colored paper is underrated; there are so many ways to stimulate participation with this basic art supply. Participants can trace their hand and cut it out or cut the paper into ribbon shapes to decorate activity rooms. Cut out leaves, hearts, pumpkins, fruits, and other objects and have participants color or write poems on them.

Tissue Paper   Tissue paper comes in all sorts of shapes, such as human figures, flowers, squares, circles, and so forth. A popular project is to cover a bottle with tissue paper and then shellac it. Another good project is to make a stained glass look-alike by first creating a frame and then pasting together sheets of tissue paper; when held up to a window, it gives the illusion of stained glass.

Kitchen Supplies to Use with TTAP

Commonly, the kitchen in any facility has more supplies than the art closet. The following is a list of common objects that can have creative uses:

Paper plates

Plastic cups

Napkins

Coffee stirrers

Plastic trays

Empty cans from soup and coffee

Plastic bags for garbage

Nursing Supplies to Use with TTAP

Nursing departments are another creative place from which to get supplies. Be sure to get permission from the proper authority to use the following items so that the safety of residents is not compromised:

Plastic cups with lids

Containers that are no longer used

Plastic sterile gloves

Plastic liners

Plastic sticks

Look in the Garbage

The old saying, "One man's trash is another man's treasure," is actually creative thinking at work. Artwork can be made from scraps of metal, old lamp parts, sticks, and large cardboard that comes from carpet rolls, just to name a few. The following are only a few examples of commonly thrown-out things that make great project materials. Find out which day of the month the large garbage is collected, and watch what can be found!

Cardboard boxes

Cardboard rolls

Lampshades and parts

Used supplies

Bags of magazines

Bags of paper

What Can Be Found for Free

Yes, free! Many stores will save commonly discarded materials for a thera-pist; just ask! The following is a list of places from which a therapist can receive free materials; store owners, organizations, and so forth feel that they are contributing to the program.

Fabric stores

Frame shops: pieces of colored paper and cardboard

Art suppliers: brushes, paints, strips of wood, cardboard

Flea markets: old toys, containers, buckets, hardware

Friends and family

Community: local women's club, garden club

Local colleges

What Can Be Found in Local Stores for Less than $10.00

Paper plates

Paper cups

Ballons

Wood sticks

Straws

Plaster

Bowls

Wooden cigar boxes

Chinese take-out boxes

Where to Get Donations

Hardware stores

Cigarette shops

Department stores

Small town shops

Frame stores

Fabric shops

Drapery stores

BASIC START-UP MATERIALS NEEDED FOR MEDITATION GROUP PROGRAM

You will need a tape or CD player and music from the six categories.

1. **Earth music**

    Albinoni: *Adagio for Strings and Organ*

    Giazotto, Conductor; Paillard Chamber Orchestra (RCA 65468-2-rc)

    Draws one into the inner world with pulling sounds; can affect the wakening of memories, yet tends to have a sad quality.

    Beethoven: *Symphony No. 7, Movement 2*

    Pablo Casals, Conductor; Marlboro Festival Orchestra, Sony Classical (SMK 45893)

    This piece often is described as music with a heartbeat. This music can awaken body responses or feelings that invite in-depth exploration.

    Vaughan Williams: *Pastoral Symphony*

    Bryden Thomson, Conductor; The London Symphony (CHAN 8594)

    This music has a sweeping effect and can be used to explore various moods; may evoke spiritual as well as emotional responses.

    Vaughan Williams: *Symphony No. 5*

    Andre Previn, Conductor; The London Symphony (RCA 60586-2RG)

    The first three movements may be used in whole or in part to evoke a long (more than 30 minutes) inner journey. Evokes depth as it leads into varying moods. Overall, it is an uplifting piece of music.

2. **Air music**

    Bach: *Orchestral Suite No. 3 in D Major, Movement 2*

    Matthias Bamert, Conductor; BBC Philharmonic (CHAN 9259)

    This is one of Bach's most famous pieces of music. It has an opening quality that stimulates imaging; it touches the soul.

Beethoven: *Symphony No. 9, Movement 1*

Eugene Ormandy, Conductor; Philadelphia Orchestra (CBS MYK 37241)

Exhilarating and vibrating sounds, this work can awaken creativity of all types. Excellent for renewing energy and rejuvenation.

Berlioz: *Symphonie Fantastique, Movement II*

Jean Martinon, Conductor; ORTF National Orchestra (EMI CZS762739-2)

This piece is described as celebratory; it is uplifting and moves into joyful sounds.

Ravel: *Introduction and Allegro*

Skaila Kanga and Academy of St. Martin-in-the-Fields, Chamber Ensemble (CHANDOS 8621)

3. **Fire music**

Bach: *Toccata and Fugue in D Minor*

Matthias Bamert, Conductor; BBC Philharmonic (CHAN 9259)

This piece evokes drama and power. Excellent to use for group work when painting or drawing.

Brahms: *Symphony No. 3 in F Major, Opus 90, Movement 1*

George Szell, Conductor; Cleveland Orchestra (CBS MYK 37777)

This piece has been described as a large container in which one feels sweeping emotions.

Bruckner: *Symphony No. 8, Movement II: Scherzo*

Sir George Solti, Conductor; Chicago Symphony Orchestra (London 430 228)

Strong sounds that lead to instant feelings that surface to the mind.

Wagner: *Flying Dutchman, Overture* and *Tannhauser, Overture*

George Szell, Conductor; Cleveland Orchestra (CBS MYK 38486)

Flying Dutchman evokes excitement and passion and fires the imagination with images. *Tannhauser* has been described as having elements of earthy and spiritual sounds. Provides a depth and richness for individuals to experience. Provides a journey toward resolution of conflict.

4.   Water music

Bartok: *Music for Strings, Percussion and Celesta, Movement 1: Andante Tranquillo*

Leonard Bernstein, Conductor; New York Philharmonic (CBS MK 42227)

Haunting music that has been described as possessing a universal quality to evoke a deep response.

Beethoven: *String Quartet in C Sharp Minor, Opus 131*

Alban Berg Quartet (EMI CDC7 47137-2)

This music has been described as having a nurturing quality. It is smooth and can bring attention to the inner child.

Brahms: *Symphony No. 2, Movement III, Andante*

George Szell, Conductor; Cleveland Orchestra (CBS MYK 337258)

This piece is uplifting and lively; it has the ability to evoke positive inner responses.

Brahms: *Symphony No. 3, Movements II and III*

This music is inspiring and uplifting and can be used to stimulate imagery.

5.   Descent music

Bach: *Come Sweet Death* and *Prelude in B Minor*

Matthias Bamert, Conductor; BBC Philharmonic (CHAN 9259)

Come Sweet Death evokes feelings of sadness. *Prelude in B Minor* is string music that has tension within the sounds. It has a deep, probing effect, so be careful when using it, because of its strong ability to stir emotions.

Beethoven: *Symphony No. 3 ''Eroica,'' Movement 2*

Sir Neville Marriner, Conductor; Academy of St. Martin-in-the-Fields (Phillips 410 044)

This piece has a slow and somber effect, which can be used in a grieving situation.

Holst: *The Planets, Saturn*

Gyorgy Ligeti, Conductor; Boston Symphony (Stereo 419 475-2)

Excellent piece for deep exploration. This piece pulls you into deep subconscious issues yet resonates with hope and resolution.

6. **Ascent music**

Bach: *Mass in B Minor, "Qui Tollis"*

Karl Richer, Conductor; Munich Bach Choir and Orchestra (Musikfest 413 688-2)

This piece has been described as inspirational, with awe and reverence.

Mahler: *Symphony No. 5, Movement III*

Sir John Barbirolli, Conductor; New Philharmonia Orchestra (EMI CDM7 69186-2)

This piece features the harp and has a true spirit of transcendence.

Mozart: *Vesperae Solennes, Laudate Dominum*

Joseph Silverstein, Conductor; Utah Symphony Orchestra with Frederica von Stade and the Mormon Tabernacle Choir (London 436 284-2)

Lifts one to inspirational heights. This piece has singing and orchestration.

BASIC START-UP MATERIALS NEEDED FOR STEP 3: MUSIC TO IMAGE

11″ × 14″ paper or 18″ × 24″ pads of white paper

11″ × 14″ paper or 18″ × 24″ pads of lower grade paper

Pastel chalks

Colored pencils

Colored markers with various tip sizes and widths

Oil crayons/pastels

Drawing pencils: HB, 2B, 3B, 6B (numbers indicate hardness of lead)

Erasers

Watercolors

Watercolor brushes (several sizes)

Plastic trays for mixing and holding water

Set of acrylic paints, brushes, disposable palettes, and canvases

Scissors

White school-grade paper glue

Glue sticks

Colored glitter or sand

BASIC START-UP MATERIALS NEEDED FOR STEP 4: FROM THE IMAGE INTO SCULPTURE

Crayola Model Magic: tubs of white, red, yellow, and blue

Omya air-dry clay

Modeling tools

Rolling pins

Clay hammers/various surfaces

Clay cutters

Clay extruding gun

Crayola fun shapes on rolling pins

Fimo (plain) & Fimo mixed color kit

Push molds

Character molds: hands, feet, heads

Sculpey modeling clay

Rigid Wrap (nontoxic wrap that contains plaster; easily molded onto all types of surfaces)

Fiberboard cones

Celluclay instant papier-mâché

Armature wire netting

Paris craft (used over wire)

Plaster of Paris

Plaster of Paris molds

Graphic Organizing Tools

DESCRIPTIVE PATTERNS

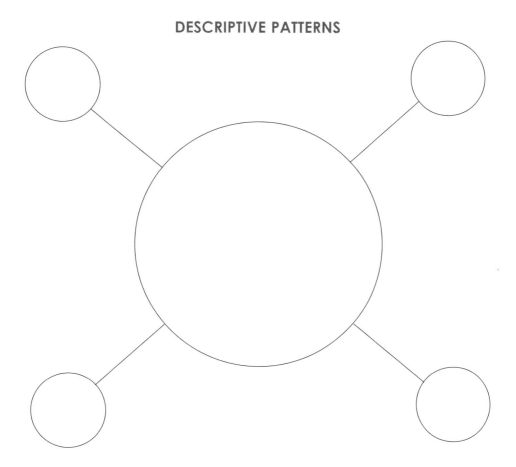

Descriptive patterns can be used to organize facts or characteristics about specific people, places, things, and events. This is the simplest form of graphic display. Each participant receives a copy to start working on a particular theme. If the chosen theme is holidays, for example, then each participant can write down the most significant four holidays that they remember. Then the therapist can display on the group chart the four most common among the group. There are many possibilities for how the group can proceed to pick one holiday to use as the theme. Another example of how this descriptive pattern chart can be used is by starting the group with music. The therapist can play a tape of nature sounds and then have a theme discussion regarding the sounds heard. Each individual can be asked to share a thought that came to mind while listening to the nature sounds. This enables each individual to describe a personal memory regarding a special moment or an event.

PROCESS AND CAUSATION PATTERNS

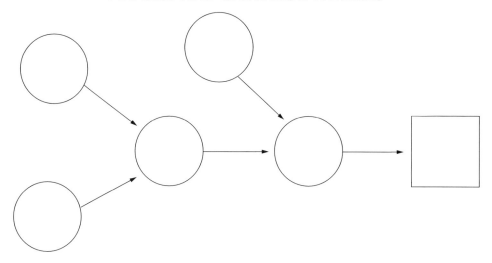

Process and causation patterns can organize information into a causal network that leads to a specific outcome or into a sequence of steps that lead to a specific product, idea, or elements of a theme. If the group has chosen making flowers as a theme for an art activity, then a process/causation chart can be used to organize the many different ways in which a flower can be made. For example, a flower can be made individually, then organized into a bunch, and then placed into an arrangement. If a therapist is working with a cognitively challenged group, then this process is crucial for visually organizing thoughts and thereby preventing frustration and anxiety.

GENERALIZATION PATTERNS

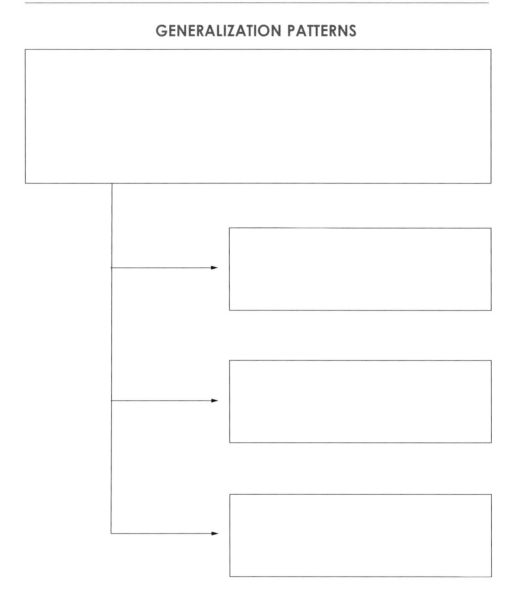

Generalization patterns organize information into generalized supporting information. This is a good diagram to use to back up theme information. This graphic organizer could be used to give examples of various cars that the clients owned or of types of trees that grow in various states.

SEQUENCE PATTERNS

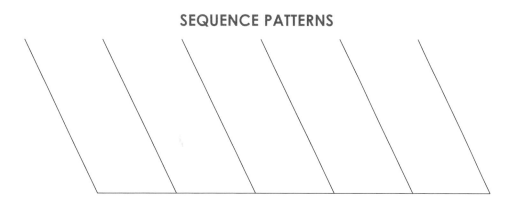

Sequence patterns organize events in a specific chronological order. If you were discussing events in history chronologically, then this would be an excellent graphic organizer. This also is an excellent cognitive tool to stimulate recall abilities.

PROBLEM-SOLVING PATTERNS

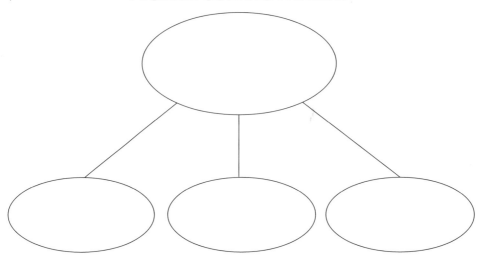

Problem-solving patterns organize information into an identified problem and its possible solutions. This is another excellent format for dealing with conflict or problems. It gives the user direction in the narrative, and it gives the participants the ability to interact and be heard. A good example of problem solving is when two people who live together cannot adjust to the living environment. This technique can enable clients to work out living arrangements by identifying what is personally important to each one individually.

CONCEPT PATTERNS

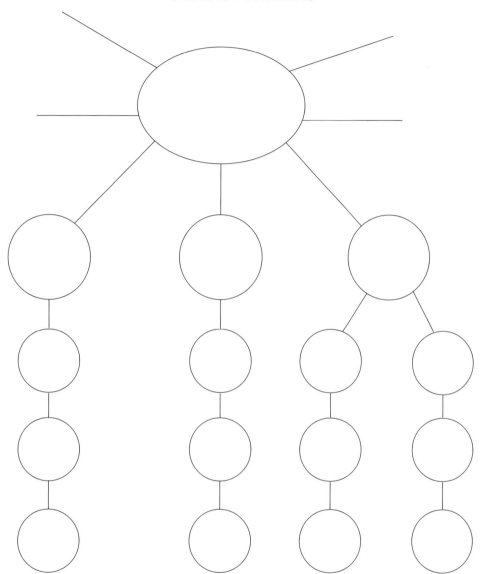

Concept patterns are the most general of all patterns. Like descriptive patterns, they deal with people, places, things, and events, but they represent an entire class or category and usually illustrate specific examples and defining characteristics of the concept. An example of using a concept pattern is to define a special evening event and all of the various foods needed.

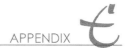

Themes in Therapeutic Thematic Arts Programming

The following themes have been developed successfully into theme programming:

changes	angels	food
symbols	life lessons	flowers
seasons	summer	family
culture	smells	jobs
systems	textures	religion
facts	fashion	holidays
communication	movies	music
languages	personalities	dances
body language	games	nations
colors	months	current events
animals	decades	women's issues
the ocean	centuries	men's issues
inventions	families	hobbies
fantasy	children	the arts
conflict	memories	the sciences
solutions	travel	the humanities
traditions	mysteries	
mountains	books	

Index

Page numbers followed by *f* indicate figures; those followed by *t* indicate tables.